THE EXPERT'S GUIDE TO WEIGHT-LOSS SURGERY

DR. GARTH DAVIS is the medical director of the Davis Clinic at the Methodist Hospital in Houston, Texas, and stars on the hit TLC show *Big Medicine*. Recently named a "Super Doc" by *Texas Monthly*, Dr. Davis lives in Houston with his family.

LAURA TUCKER has coauthored books on a wide range of topics. She lives in Brooklyn, New York, with her husband and daughter.

THE EXPERT'S GUIDE TO

WEIGHT-LOSS SURGERY

||||||||||||||||||||||||||||||||||||||||||||||||||||||||||||||||||||||||||||||||

Is it right for me?

What happens during surgery?

How do I keep the weight off?

GARTH DAVIS, M.D.

STAR OF TLC'S

BIG MEDICINE

WITH LAURA TUCKER

A PLUME BOOK

PLUME
Published by the Penguin Group
Penguin Group (USA) Inc., 375 Hudson Street, New York, New York 10014, U.S.A. • Penguin Group (Canada), 90 Eglinton Avenue East, Suite 700, Toronto, Ontario, Canada M4P 2Y3 (a division of Pearson Penguin Canada Inc.) • Penguin Books Ltd, 80 Strand, London WC2R 0RL, England • Penguin Ireland, 25 St. Stephen's Green, Dublin 2, Ireland (a division of Penguin Books Ltd.) • Penguin Group (Australia), 250 Camberwell Road, Camberwell, Victoria 3124, Australia (a division of Pearson Australia Group Pty. Ltd.) • Penguin Books India Pvt. Ltd., 11 Community Centre, Panchsheel Park, New Delhi – 110 017, India • Penguin Group (NZ), 67 Apollo Drive, Rosedale, North Shore 0632, New Zealand (a division of Pearson New Zealand Ltd.) • Penguin Books (South Africa) (Pty.) Ltd., 24 Sturdee Avenue, Rosebank, Johannesburg 2196, South Africa

Penguin Books Ltd., Registered Offices: 80 Strand, London WC2R 0RL, England

First published by Plume, a member of Penguin Group (USA) Inc. Previously published in a Hudson Street Press edition.

First Plume Printing, March 2010
10 9 8 7 6 5 4 3 2 1

Ⓟ REGISTERED TRADEMARK—MARCA REGISTRADA

The Library of Congress has catalogued the Hudson Street Press edition as follows:
Davis, Garth, Dr.
   The expert's guide to weight-loss surgery : is it right for me? what happens during surgery? how do I keep the weight off? / Dr. Garth Davis, with Laura Tucker.
     p.   cm.
   Includes bibliographical references and indexes.
   ISBN 978-1-59463-052-1 (hc.)
   ISBN 978-0-452-29606-0 (pbk.)
   1. Obesity—Surgery.   2. Weight loss.   3. Gastrointestinal system—Surgery.   4. Gastric bypass.
   I. Tucker, Laura, 1973–   II. Title.
   RD540.D18 2009
   617.4'3—dc22   2008034239

Printed in the United States of America
Set in Fairfield Light

PUBLISHER'S NOTE
Neither the publisher nor the authors are engaged in rendering professional advice or services to the individual reader. The ideas, procedures, and suggestions contained in this book are not intended as a substitute for consulting with your physician. All matters regarding your health require medical supervision. Neither the authors nor the publisher shall be liable or responsible for any loss or damage allegedly arising from any information or suggestion in this book.

I dedicate this book, with utmost respect, to my father, Robert Davis. It was always a dream of mine to grow up to be like him, and I am still striving to do so. It is an amazing honor to be his partner, and it has cemented our relationship, not only as father and son, but also as the best of friends. Neither this book nor the wonderful weight-loss program we have set up in Houston would be possible without him.

Contents

Acknowledgments

I would like to acknowledge first and foremost the many people who have given me the chance to help them. I know that the struggles and triumphs presented in this book are just the tip of the iceberg compared to what they go through on a daily basis. I am honored that they trust me to care for them, and I thank them for allowing me to share in their joy and success.

I would also like to thank all the invaluable team members who have helped me create and continue such a wonderful weight-loss program. Sue Thompson, Kathie Nelson, and Karin Larson-Pollock have created an amazing weight-loss program at the Methodist Hospital, and Trudy Ivins single-handedly brought to life a center of excellence in bariatrics at University General Hospital. Our very large program requires quite a bit of coordination, so I must thank Allison Skelton, Zola Landers, and Tara Corbett for their dedication and support. The dieticians in our program are crucial to its success, so I am grateful to Kathryn Lito, Jennifer Naples, and Stephanie Barrocas for all their hard work in helping my patients reach their goals.

Diet and surgery are only part of a successful weight-loss team. I am therefore indebted to Mary Jo Rapini for all the hard work she has put into our program, this book and for costarring on *Big Medicine* with me. I consider her to be an invaluable part of our success—both my own and the patients I treat. I also would like to thank Monica Agosta, Stephen Morris, and Deborah Lindeen, who also have played such important roles in the mental health of my patients.

I am always impressed at Austin Davis's dedication to our program. Besides helping me with this book, he regularly attends our support groups and has selflessly taught many of my patients who had never exercised before the true meaning of what it means to be fit.

I must also thank my truly amazing office staff. Jamie Carr is one of the most experienced and well-known bariatric nurses in the country. I cannot thank her enough, not only for helping me with this book, but also for agreeing to become a part of this team and helping me both create and lead the program. I must also thank Kimberly Taylor, who was invaluable in helping me with this book, and with my office; her professionalism and dedication are much appreciated. I could go on forever, so let me just give a huge thanks to Melinda, Alma, Zintia, Maria, Tammy, Melissa, Tameki, Becky, Tricia, and Ellen. I appreciate you all more than you know.

I never could have written this book without the help of Laura Tucker. I was absolutely amazed that after spending just a few days with me she was able to learn not just about the weight-loss surgeries but also the plight of the obese patients. She is a fantastic writer, and I thank her dearly for her patience and her help in writing this book.

I'd also like to thank the amazing team at Hudson Street Press for their professionalism, particularly Luke Dempsey for his continued faith in me and in the project, and Danielle Friedman for her sensitivity, guidance, and meticulous attention to detail.

I must thank my loving family for all their support. To my sisters, Toni and Kim, who have always been so loving and supportive, and to my always doting and caring mother, Arlene, thank you so much for all of your care and love. And to my brother-in-law, Paul, who handled the amazing number of legal issues that go into writing a book, and who is always watching my back. Finally, I would like to thank Kelly, my wife, who is so patient with my long hours, and who truly is my partner in life, and my sweet baby, Avery, who is my motivation.

Introduction

"I look down at my body and think, "How did I get to be like this? I'm trapped in here; it's like a prison."

"It is not an exaggeration to say that I have felt guilty and anxious about every single bite of food that has passed my lips in the last thirty years."

"I see how happy and confident and sexy other women look. I see the attention they attract, the fun they have showing off their clothes and their bodies, and the voice inside my head says, 'That's not for you. That has never been for you, and it will never be for you.'

"There is no diet I haven't tried. Low-carb, no-carb, all-carb, low-fat, no-fat, 'good' fat. WeightWatchers, Jenny Craig, Quick Weight Loss, grapefruit, cabbage—you name it, I've starved myself on it. Do I lose? Sure I do. Do I gain it back? Every time, plus some for good measure."

Do any of these sentiments sound familiar to you? If they do, then you're probably struggling with the disease called obesity. You're not alone; millions of Americans are right there with you, and those numbers are increasing every year. And if you heard your own voice in the statements above, then you're reading the right book.

The simple fact is that obesity is a disease, and an inherited one. Most of the population doesn't realize this. In fact, many *doctors* don't realize this, which is why the prevailing medical advice to people struggling with the disease of obesity continues to be "eat less, and exercise more."

The problem with that advice, as you probably know all too well, is that *it doesn't work*. Do diet and exercise play a role in how much you weigh? Sure. In fact, as we'll discuss at greater length later, the role they play is an important one. But the fact remains that most people who rely on diet and exercise alone to control obesity will fail.

Diet and exercise alone are overwhelmingly
unsuccessful interventions for the obese.

So too many people with this disease go untreated—and with severe consequences to their health. Living with obesity means more than simply coping with a compromised quality of life and poor self-esteem; it often means living with painful chronic diseases, such as arthritis, and potentially fatal ones, such as heart disease and diabetes. In fact, obesity is currently poised to outstrip cigarette smoking as the single leading cause of preventable disease in the United States.

It doesn't have to be this way. There is a solution—one that can help you not only shed pounds and the health risks associated with obesity but also calm your hunger and normalize your relationship with food. That solution, and whether or not it's the right one for you, is the subject of this book.

My name is Garth Davis, and I'm a weight-loss surgeon in Houston, Texas. You may have seen me and my father, Dr. Robert Davis, on our TLC show, *Big Medicine*. The response to the show has been a little overwhelming—neither one of us ever thought we'd be recognized in airports!—but it also has been tremendously gratifying. We agreed to do the show in the first place because we wanted to give our patients a voice, something that is too often denied to the obese. We wanted to show the realities of weight-loss surgery—the good as well as the bad—without media sensationalism. Most of all, we wanted to show that while surgery might not be the right choice for everyone, if it is the right choice for you, it can truly change your life.

Writing this book is part of that same effort. *Big Medicine* has increased people's awareness about the surgeries, and I believe it has raised the level of discourse about them. But from my perspective, the real by-product of the show has been more questions. When people come over to me in an airport, they don't want an autograph or a picture; they want me to tell them whether I think they're a good candidate for the surgery, or they want to ask my opinion about which type of surgery—the band or the bypass, for example—is likely to be most successful for them. Some of them already have had weight-loss surgery, and they want to know which vitamins we recommend to our patients, or they want to know how to cope now that their weight loss has stalled. Others want to know where they can go to find support, now that all the weight is gone but the painful feelings left over from years of obesity are still there.

This book is my attempt to answer these questions. Because our practice specializes in weight-loss surgery, we've seen and heard it all—or most of it, anyway. I'm not just talking about the newest surgical technologies and techniques, but also the anecdotal tips and tricks that can make the procedures themselves easier and the aftermath more enjoyable and more successful. I know, from my own patients and from *Big Medicine*, that there are a lot of people who are hungry for that information. Indeed, much of my own knowledge comes from listening to my patients, whose funny, generous, honest voices you will find throughout this book. Thanks to them, I am a student every day.

A few caveats before we begin. Much of the advice you'll find in these pages has to do with the way we do things in *our* practice and in *our* clinic. I have some pretty strong opinions about these surgeries, developed over the many years I've been doing them and the more than 1,000 surgeries I've performed. Some of those thoughts aren't the "party line." I'd advise you to take your own search for a doctor pretty seriously (I'll show you how to do just that in Chapter 6), and then listen to what he or she says. Use this book as a guide and a prompt to ask questions and to do additional research, but remember that your own doctor's advice and recommendations should—must—always trump the advice you'll find here.

That said, here's what you'll find in the pages that follow. First, I want to talk about the factors contributing to the obesity epidemic, and why your weight control issues aren't entirely your fault—refreshing news to some of you, I'm sure! Then we'll take a closer look at the different types of surgery available and the strengths and problems associated with each. Just as I do with my patients, I'll give you the information you need to determine if surgery is right for you—and if so, which one. I'll help you to find a good surgeon and to navigate the murky waters of the insurance process, which often can be one of the most trying parts of this journey.

And because it's all about long-term success, we'll not only talk about diet and exercise after surgery but also what to expect from your emotions— both during the euphoric "honeymoon" phase and beyond. The surgery isn't a cure for a disordered relationship with food, so we'll talk about how to arrive at a healthier understanding with yourself and with your plate. And I'll give you proven strategies to help you negotiate some of the most common pitfalls my patients face.

Weight-loss surgery isn't a magic bullet. It won't "cure" everything that's wrong with you, and it does carry risks. But it can be a very effective tool to combat the disease of obesity, particularly if you're committed to change and have lots of support. I have tried to make this book as comprehensive as possible, and it is my hope that it can be one of those supports for you.

From my experience, the voices at the beginning of this chapter are typical of those living with this disease. My patients aren't lazy people or people who just haven't yet tried the right diet. They're not ignorant, and they didn't find their way to morbid obesity simply because they were lacking in willpower. But by the time they get to me—after a lifetime of secret shame, of whispers and stares, and of diet failure after diet failure—they often think that the way they feel is the way it's always going to be.

That's just not the truth. I've seen patients smile and show off bodies they've felt sick about since childhood. I've looked through wedding albums of patients who thought they'd never date; I've held the babies of people who, before surgery, thought they'd always be infertile. Seeing patient after patient changed, both physically and emotionally, by this tool is one of the great pleasures of my job.

This journey isn't for everyone, and it's not an easy path; in order to be successful, a great deal will be required of you. But, as you will see in the pages that follow, this is an intervention that has worked for hundreds of thousands of people, and it is one that can work for you.

My simple wish is that, after reading this book, you will understand that the way you feel right now doesn't need to be the way you feel forever. Take heart: You're not alone, and there *is* hope.

The Expert's Guide to
Weight-Loss
Surgery

CHAPTER ONE

The Costs of Obesity

"Eventually my grandkids just stopped asking me to play. They knew I couldn't make it to the park, let alone chase them while we were there."

"Being obese meant that I didn't go to my daughter's high school graduation lunch because I didn't want to embarrass her."

"For me being obese means knowing I'm going to die too young, like my mom did."

It's widely held that obesity is the last bastion of acceptable prejudice in our culture. Can you imagine people openly laughing at a person with any other disability or a legislator proposing, as one did in Mississippi in 2008, to forbid restaurants from serving someone with any other disease?

As far as I'm concerned, the costs of obesity cannot be overestimated. And these costs increase as the number of obese people in this country grow, as they do every year. Some of these costs are quantifiable; others, like the time you might have spent playing with your grandchildren, are not.

In this chapter, I'd like to take a closer look at what it means to be obese. First, we'll define what exactly obesity means, and then we'll look at some of the costs—financial, physical, social, and otherwise—associated with this disease.

Defining Our Terms

"I couldn't believe it when the word obese *came out of my doctor's mouth. I'd always been heavy, but I couldn't believe I was obese."*

Obesity isn't just a schoolyard taunt; it's a medical term used to describe a high degree of body fat. Doctors use a tool called the Body Mass Index (BMI), a ratio of weight to height, to assess a person's weight and risk for chronic disease. Doctors generally consider people with a BMI of 30 or over to be obese.

In this book, we're going to concern ourselves primarily with the category of morbid obesity, which is defined by the National Institutes of Health (NIH) as:

- Being 100 pounds or more over your ideal body weight, or having a BMI over 40, or

- Having a BMI of 35 or greater and one or more co-morbid conditions. Co-morbidities are the diseases or conditions caused by obesity, and there are a lot of them. (More on this shortly.)

There are three ways to calculate your BMI:

1) You can use one of the many BMI calculators on the Internet, such as the one offered by the National Heart, Lung, and Blood Institute (NHLBI) here: nhlbisupport.com/bmi/

2) If you like math or are curious about how doctors get to this number, you can get out your pen and paper and calculate your BMI by yourself. Here's the equation:

Weight in Pounds

÷

((Height in inches)×(Height in inches))×703

So a person who is 5 feet 9 inches and weighs 300 pounds has a BMI of 44. Here's that math:

300 divided by (69×69)×703=44.29

3) Or you can find your BMI using the chart on page 273.

What it means:

If your BMI is:

Less than 18.5, you're considered underweight.
Between 18.5 and 24.9, you're considered a normal weight.
Between 25 and 29.9, you're considered overweight.
Between 30 and 34.9, you're considered obese.
Between 35 and 50, you're considered morbidly obese.
Over 50, you're considered extremely obese, or super-obese.

Good to know: BMI isn't a perfect measurement. A simple height-to-weight ratio doesn't take into consideration how that weight is distributed or what it's made of. For instance, muscle weighs considerably more than fat, which means that most bodybuilders at the height of their powers probably would record as close to obese. Similarly, people who have very little muscle mass (something we see quite commonly in the elderly) may not show up as overweight at all if their BMI is the only measure applied—even if they have a dangerous amount of excess fat. If there's any question, your doctor can use more sophisticated techniques to determine whether or not you are obese.

Finally, where the fat is distributed on your body may actually be more important than your BMI in determining how dangerous your weight is to your health. Doctors use what's called a waist-to-hip ratio to determine the danger you're in, and cardiac researchers have shown that it's a better predictor of heart attack risk than BMI.

To simplify, there are two basic body types: apple and pear. Apples have big (usually hard) bellies, accompanied by skinnier arms and legs. A pear-shaped person usually has a softer abdomen and a bigger lower half—a large bottom and heavy legs. Men are usually apple-shaped, and women are usually pears—although this isn't always the case.

Unfortunately, the abdominal fat carried by the apple shape is a danger sign. I have treated pear-shaped women who weighed 400 pounds and had

BMIs in the 60s—and yet who did not have a single health problem and took no medications at all. On the other hand, I often see apple-shaped men with comparatively low BMIs—in the 30s, say—who already suffer from diabetes, high blood pressure, high cholesterol, and heart disease. So you may want to talk to your doctor about whether your particular body type puts your health at special risk.

You're Not Alone

So now we know what obesity is. But because obesity is such an isolating disease by its very nature, you may not know how many people are suffering right alongside you. I do, because my waiting room is filled with people just like you every single day.

The statistics are staggering. And the most frightening part is that these numbers are increasing with every passing year.

Consider the following:

- 61 percent of Americans are either overweight or obese. According to the Centers for Disease Control and Prevention, in 2001, 44 million Americans—approximately one in five—were considered obese. It is estimated that between 10 and 20 million are morbidly obese.

- In 2006, more than 20 percent of the population in forty-six out of the fifty states was obese.

- The United States isn't the only country with a problem. The World Health Organization (WHO) estimated in 2005 that more than approximately 1.6 billion adults (age fifteen-plus) were overweight worldwide, and at least 400 million adults were obese.

Even more alarming, the statistics show us that those numbers are growing at a steady clip:

- The National Health and Nutrition Examination Survey (NHANES) showed that obesity increased from 15 to 33 percent of adults between 1960 and 1994.

- There was a 400 percent increase in obesity among children during that same time, with the result that 18.8 percent of children are now obese. Children are the fastest growing obese population; it is estimated that one in every three children growing up in the United States today is obese. These are especially chilling statistics, given that 80 percent of obese children become obese adults.

- According to the CDC report, the obesity rate has increased by 74 percent since 1991. Researchers now believe that in just a few short years, the entire Southeast will have obesity rates greater than 35 percent, and the rest of the country is not far behind.

The term *obesity epidemic*, then, is not an exaggeration. And, as we will see, the costs of this epidemic are considerable.

The Costs of Obesity

In this section, I'd like to review some of the costs of this obesity epidemic. These costs are vast, and their consequences far-reaching, but they continue to be undervalued, in my opinion—even by people who live every day with this disease.

Economic

> *"I know that I've lost accounts because people think that some-one who looks like me must be lazy and unmotivated."*

It's estimated that in 2001, Americans spent between 100 and 120 billion dollars a year on health care directly related to the obesity epidemic, which accounted for more than 9 percent of the nation's health-care expenditures. That report, issued by the Surgeon General, concluded that "obesity is among the most pressing health-care challenges we are facing today."

Obese people suffer terribly from the economic impact of their disease. It costs a lot to be sick all the time! And Americans spend an additional 40 billion dollars on so-called treatments—diets and diet products—that don't work.

Prejudice against obese people in the workplace—which, unfortunately, is very real—accounts for other economic costs. The American Obesity Association looked at twenty-nine field and laboratory studies, for instance, and found that overweight people were overwhelmingly subject to discrimination in appraisals of their performance and other workplace criteria.[*] Not only are the wages of the morbidly obese dramatically lower,[†] but other studies have shown that weight is a bigger variable in the decision to hire than anything else. Another study showed that people display more negative attitudes toward overweight employees than they do toward ex-felons or ex–mental patients.[‡]

We hear these stories every day in our practice. One of my father's patients watched her thinner, less qualified colleagues accept promotions at her high-powered law firm for years while she wilted on the vine. A year later—and 100 pounds lighter—she's now the managing director of the firm. Hers is ultimately a success story, but many aren't. Even school is harder for obese people. More than one of my patients has told me about the discomfort of squeezing into a desk in a seminar; another dropped out of college completely after the chair she was sitting on in a lecture hall collapsed.

In what ways—from expensive medications to missed work opportunities—has obesity cost you?

Social

> *"The stares. The giggles. The comments they think you can't hear. The fear that something will happen, bringing even more attention to your size. It's just so much easier to stay home."*

Have you ever turned down an invitation or a social opportunity simply because you felt self-conscious?

I'd be very surprised if your answer was no. Practically every one of my

---

[*] M. Roehling, "Weight-Based Discrimination in Employment: Psychological and Legal Aspects," *Personnel Psychology*, 1999, 52, 969–1016.

[†] Charles L. Baum and William F. Ford, "The Wage Effects of Obesity: A Longitudinal Study," *Health Economics*, 2004, 13, no. 9.

[‡] M. Roehling, "Weight Discrimination in the American Workplace: Ethical Issues and Analysis," *Journal of Business Ethics*, 2002, vol. 40, no. 2.

patients eventually mentions the much-dreaded high-school reunion. There is no question that excess weight can prevent you from living your life as fully as you might like to.

You've probably also said no to some events for logistical reasons or because you didn't want to have to deal with the shame of having to ask for a seat-belt extension or the discomfort of wondering if you'd be able to fit into the booth at a restaurant. The company trip to the amusement park isn't such a relaxing morale booster if you can't be sure you'll be allowed on the rides, is it?

It may be harder to track these costs than the economic ones we've discussed or the physical ones I'll get to in a minute. But to my mind, they're no less significant for being harder to quantify—and they may be the most painful ones of all.

Physical

> *"My diabetes was totally uncontrolled, and finally, after we'd tried everything, my doctor said it straight out: 'If you don't lose weight, you're going to be dead in five years.'"*

We call the physical consequences of obesity co-morbidities. At best, these co-morbidities threaten your quality of life, as you know all too well. Eventually they will threaten your life itself. Mortality is dramatically increased in obese people; in fact, a BMI of greater than 32 is associated with a *doubled* risk of premature death. This correlation to mortality is actually how the World Health Organization decided to draw distinctions between the overweight, obese, morbidly obese, and super-obese BMI categories; each time the mortality stats jumped, they started a new category.

Based on the science, I feel very confident saying that, on average, being obese takes ten years or more off your life.

Obesity is absolutely a life-threatening condition, as it wreaks havoc on many of the body's systems.

Unfortunately, many of the co-morbidities listed here will be familiar to you; if they're not conditions you already live with, they undoubtedly loom on the horizon. Putting them together this way demonstrates very clearly how obesity jeopardizes every one of the body's systems. Let's take a look:

Cardiovascular disease. This is the number-one killer of Americans. Being overweight is a major (and some doctors would say *the* major) risk factor for heart disease.

Being obese is also associated with other risk factors of heart disease, such as high LDL "bad" cholesterol, lower HDL "good" cholesterol, high triglycerides, and high blood pressure.

Type 2 diabetes. Diabetes is the body's inability to regulate its own blood sugar. It is strongly correlated to being overweight: According to the National Institute of Diabetes and Digestive and Kidney Diseases, more than 85 percent of people with type 2 diabetes are overweight. Because of this correlation, we are seeing staggering increases in diabetes in this country—what amounts to a diabetes epidemic—that has everything to do with the rise in obesity.

Diabetes is not only expensive and difficult to manage; it also comes with a whole range of possible complications—including heart disease, high blood pressure, blindness, nerve damage, and kidney damage. More than 60 percent of nontraumatic lower-limb amputations occur in people with diabetes.

Hypertension (high blood pressure). Hypertension is a leading cause of heart disease and stroke—the first and third leading causes of death in this country. Being obese more than doubles your risk that you'll suffer from what doctors call the silent killer. And the more obese you are, the more likely it is that you'll have it.

Cancer. This one surprises a lot of people, but a recent paper published in the *Journal of the American Medical Association* claimed that 90,000 deaths from cancer in the United States could be prevented every year if Americans kept their BMIs normal (at 25).

There is a three to four times increased risk of endometrial or ovarian cancer in the obese, and being obese doubles your risk of breast cancer. Cancer of the kidney, colon and rectum, esophagus, prostate, and gallbladder have also been linked to obesity, and scientists believe that many other cancers are linked as well.

Sleep apnea. Apnea means "without breath" in Greek; people with this condition actually stop breathing while they are asleep. In overweight people, this is usually because the soft tissue at the back of the throat collapses and causes an obstruction.

The obvious problem with sleep apnea is that your sleep is fragmented and disrupted. Exhaustion caused by poor sleep is a risk in its own right, of course: Car crashes and job-related accidents skyrocket in people with sleep apnea. And to make matters worse, poor sleep is strongly correlated to weight gain. Sleep apnea is also linked to impotence, memory problems, and headaches—untreated, it can cause high blood pressure and cardiovascular disease.

Gastroesophageal reflux disease (GERD). Acid reflux disease, or GERD, results when too much fat presses on the stomach, essentially pushing it up into the chest and disrupting the sphincter, which normally stops stomach acid from coming back up into the throat, so that acid floods the esophagus and burns the lining.

GERD is very painful and can cause complications such as coughing, inflammation of the esophagus, difficulty swallowing, and even esophageal cancer.

Asthma. Asthma is defined as an inflammation of the airways, causing chest tightness and difficulty breathing. Studies show that obese patients are more likely to have bad asthma, and to have it over a longer period of time. This can also be due to the reflux; acid can get into the lungs and cause inflammation. A severe asthma attack can result in death.

Gout. Gout is a very painful swelling in the joints, caused when the kidneys fail to rid the body of uric acid through the urine. It is commonly found in obese patients.

Gallbladder disease. Gallstones are balls of hardened cholesterol in the gallbladder. If they move out of the gallbladder, they can block the normal passage of bile from the liver, causing inflammation and infection. The movement of these gallstones is extremely painful, and without treatment they can lead to serious problems. Obesity is a major risk factor for gallbladder disease.

Liver disease. A buildup of fat in the liver can lead to severe liver damage, similar to what happens in the livers of alcoholics—even if you don't drink.

Although alcohol-related liver disease gets more publicity and attention, fat-related liver disease is actually the leading cause of abnormal liver function tests in the United States. These abnormal liver function tests are the result of steatohepatitis, an inflammatory liver disease, which can be followed by cirrhosis, an irreversible and deadly scarring of the liver.

Vein disease. The pressure of a large belly can cause the veins of the legs to swell, breaking the valves that prevent the blood from pooling in the legs, resulting in varicose veins. Since the obese are more prone to blood clots because of inflammatory chemicals that are released by the fat cells, this situation puts the obese at high risk for major clots in the legs, called deep vein thrombosis. If a clot breaks free, it can end up in the lungs, a condition called a pulmonary embolism, which can be fatal.

Arthritis and joint disease. The body isn't designed to support the weight of a morbidly obese person, and the joints literally get ground down and wear out as a result. Being overweight puts tremendous stress on your back, hips, knees, and ankles.

Arthritis also contributes to other co-morbidities; it is a good example of the kind of co-morbidity cascade that happens so often with obesity. If you wear your joints down, it will be very painful to exercise; and not exercising, of course, contributes to further weight gain. You may need to get your joint replaced, but it can be difficult to find an orthopedist willing to do a knee or hip replacement on a morbidly obese person. Artificial joints simply aren't designed to carry that kind of weight, and there's a higher rate of failure associated with these procedures in the morbidly obese. But without the replacement, you'll eventually find it difficult even to walk, which will put you in a wheelchair—and dramatically increase your risk of a blood clot.

Polycystic ovarian syndrome (PCOS). PCOS is a disruption in the hormonal cycle that may affect menstrual cycles and threaten fertility.

Typically estrogen is stored and broken down in the fat cells. In the obese, however, it is broken down inappropriately and turned into a testosterone-like substance, which may give rise to some of the symptoms of PCOS. These symptoms include pelvic pain, cysts on the ovaries, hair loss, acne, and increased body and facial hair. It is the most commonly diagnosed hormonal disease in reproductive-age women, and the majority of women diagnosed with this disease are either overweight or obese.

Fertility and pregnancy complications. Obesity is a significant contributor to fertility difficulties, for both men and women.

The increased estrogen we find in obese men can lead to impotence, low sperm count, and decreased libido. And fat, particularly abdominal fat, sends out hormones that can interrupt the ordinary workings of the female reproductive system. A Dutch study published in the *Journal of the American Medical Association* found that an obese woman's likelihood of conceiving decreases steadily as her BMI increases; for every BMI unit increase over 30, there was a 4 percent decrease in the rate at which participants conceived.

Pseudotumors (pseudotumor cerebri). These severe headaches are the result of increased pressure in the head. The majority of people with this condition are overweight women of childbearing age. The precise cause for the condition is unknown, but it is believed that being overweight increases pressure in the brain, leading to terrible headaches and even blindness.

Stress urinary incontinence. This is the incontinence that causes you to leak a little when you laugh or cough or get up out of a chair. Being overweight increases the stress on your bladder and the muscles around it. Obese women are nearly twice (1.7 times) as likely to suffer from urinary incontinence than are women of a normal weight.

Carpal tunnel syndrome. There's a four-times increase in the pain and weakness in the hands, known as carpal tunnel syndrome, among obese patients. Excess fat puts extra pressure on the nerves of the hand.

Dermatitis. Obese people often suffer breakdowns in the places where skin rubs together. These breakdowns are not only painful, but they can lead to serious infection.

It's a horrifying laundry list. Most of the people who walk into my office for the first time suffer not from one or two, but a combination of these co-morbidities. They live—as you might, too—with chronic pain, multiple medications, and the knowledge that each of these conditions will get worse and harder to control the more weight you carry.

It's important to realize just how serious this disease can be if it's left untreated: According to the Surgeon General's office, obesity is the preventable cause of 300,000 deaths every year in this country.

It's really quite simple:

As BMI increases, so do years of life lost.

A recent study showed that a BMI of over 35 leads to a doubling of all causes of death. Hippocrates knew this—he observed that "sudden death is more common in those who are naturally fat than in the lean" in the fourth century B.C. Insurance companies have known it for years, too. But what is fascinating to me—and we'll talk about this at much greater length in a minute—is the word *preventable*. The majority of these conditions can be reversed—*simply by losing the weight*.

In the last ten years, we've come to a greater understanding of obesity, which has contributed to our understanding of why obese people get so very sick. First of all, we're learning that fat cells aren't just storage containers holding energy we're sacking away for later. Fat actually acts like an endocrine organ, like a pancreas or an ovary, which means that our fat cells secrete inflammatory messengers—including some that cause or exacerbate diabetes and hypertension and increase cholesterol, coronary artery disease, infertility, fatty liver disease, and gallstones. The more fat you have, the more of these messengers you're making, which is part of the reason why overweight and obese people are at such risk for these diseases.

And yet the majority of the time, this potentially fatal disease goes untreated. Can you imagine a doctor dismissing someone with any other disease with advice to take a pill that has only a 3 percent chance of working? That's precisely what happens every time an obese person is sent away with the advice to "eat less and exercise." The studies vary, but conventional weight-loss approaches in the obese have been shown to fail *somewhere between 95 and 97 percent of the time.*

This, then, is another hidden cost of obesity: Appropriate-quality medical care is too often denied to the obese.

Many doctors simply find themselves frustrated by some conditions specific to the obese, such as skin breakdowns and leg swelling; they just don't know what to do. And, unfortunately, many doctors harbor the same prejudices against the obese held by the general population; the difference is that in a medical scenario, those prejudices can directly affect the type of care that obese patients receive. One of my patients told me that when she got too heavy for the conventional scale in her doctor's office, the nurse took her down to the hospital's loading dock to use the scale there. I've heard of doctors recommending that patients stop by feed lots or veterinary offices to get their weight checked. I'm not suggesting that every family doc invest in a bariatric scale—although with 60 percent of the country overweight and more than 30 percent obese, it wouldn't be a bad idea. But every doctor should be able to refer bariatric patients to a practice that is qualified to handle their care ethically and with respect.

It's not surprising, then, for my father and me to see people who haven't been to their primary care doctor in years, even when they're living in considerable pain—who would voluntarily sign up for that kind of humiliation? And so one of the populations that is most likely to need high-quality medical care often goes without that care.

Not surprisingly, the disconnect between the problem and a viable solution is making this epidemic worse. But in order to arrive at something better, we first need to have a better understanding of the root causes of obesity.

CHAPTER TWO

||||||||||||||||||||||||||||||||||||||||||||||||||||

How We Got Here—

And Why What We're Doing Now Isn't Working

"I eat more than other people because I'm hungrier than other people."

"'Put down the fork and step away from the table,' my husband tells me. Does he really think this hasn't occurred to me?"

"There's a difference between hunger and 'head' hunger. Unfortunately, I haven't exactly been able to figure out what that difference is."

Ask most doctors, and they'll tell you that the answer to obesity is diet and exercise. "Have you dieted? Try eating less," one doctor told one of my patients—someone who attended her first WeightWatchers meeting at the ripe old age of nine. The list of diets she's been on in the last thirty years takes up a full, single-spaced page. And yet the doctor had nothing more to recommend to her than what she'd always tried.

I believe that one of the reasons we've failed so badly at addressing the obesity epidemic is because the majority opinion has stuck with a misconception for far too long. I can tell you one thing for sure:

If it was as simple as "eat less and exercise,"
we would not have an obesity epidemic.

The prejudice against obesity, and the treatments recommended to address it, will only change when the medical community and society at large accepts a more sophisticated understanding of what's behind this disease.

It is my firm belief that unless we unhitch our understanding of this disease from the mistaken belief that obese people have made a lifestyle choice and just need to stop eating, we will never be able to help anyone keep the weight off for good.

Obesity: A Multifactorial Stew

Scientists call obesity "multifactorial in origin," which is to say that there are a number of factors, working together, that contribute to the disease. These factors include various genetic, environmental, and psychological causes.

**A number of factors determine whether (or not)
someone becomes obese.**

While we *can* control some of these factors, we can't control all of them. I hope that just hearing this lifts some of the weight off your shoulders. Contrary to what you may have been told your whole life, your obesity is not entirely your fault. And the reason that the diets you've been on haven't worked wasn't entirely due to your lack of willpower, either.

In fact, researchers now have the science to back up a conclusion that you probably could have reached by looking around your Thanksgiving table: that there is a strong genetic component to obesity.

Gina Kolata is a writer for the *New York Times* and the author of a book I highly recommend, called *Rethinking Thin*. In it, she cites a number of fascinating studies that go a long way toward explaining why people are obese—and why conventional diets don't work. For instance, researchers have found that skinny people fed tons and tons of calories don't get fat—they get sick. But obese people, when put on a reduced-calorie diet, develop a type of psychosis about food, clinically similar to post-traumatic stress disorder. They dream about it, hide food, binge, and think about suicide.

And it's not just in their heads, either. Obese individuals actually burn calories more slowly, which is why they require less food to maintain their weight. An experiment that severely reduced calories in obese subjects found that, even on a drastically low 450 calories a day, participants lost only 6 percent of their body weight because their metabolic rate had slowed to a crawl. Despite their weight, their bodies interpreted the reduction in calories as a threat to their continued survival.

**From a metabolic perspective, obese people on a
diet are actually starving.**

In study after study, nature trumps nurture. An article published in the *American Journal of Clinical Nutrition* focused on a study done by a group of British researchers who looked at 5,000 pairs of twins between the ages of eight and eleven—both identical twins, who share all their genes, and nonidentical twins, who share only half. They found that the differences in the children's BMIs and waist circumference were 77 percent attributable to genes. This put weight on par with height as one of the two most heritable traits.

In another study, researchers looked at husbands and wives. If a guy was overweight, was his wife overweight, too? They expected there to be a pretty close correlation; after all, husbands and wives live together, raid the same kitchen cabinets, eat a lot of meals together, and share a food culture. But that's not what they found; in fact, there was only a 10 percent correlation between a person's obesity and that of their spouse's.

When they looked at each spouse's respective gene pools, however, they saw something very different. There was a 15 percent correlation between obesity in first cousins and a 25 percent correlation between parents and children. And one Dutch study looked at twins who had been separated at birth and raised in different homes. Researchers found that even when the environments had been completely different, if one twin was obese, there was an astonishing 88 *percent* chance that the other one would be, too.

**The more genetic material shared,
the more likely there is to be a correlation
of obesity.**

We're not completely sure how the genetic mechanism works to cause obesity because this science is in its infancy, but great strides are being made every year. We do know that there is a weight at which your body feels comfortable, called a set point, and it is likely genetically determined.

Can you diet to a weight below your set point? Sure. But it's as if there's an elastic band attached to your set point, which explains why dieting is so rarely successful over the long term. Your body believes that your survival depends on you returning to that set point, so it decreases your metabolism, slowing the rate at which you burn calories, and increases your appetite, encouraging you to take in more energy in the form of calories. The more weight you lose, the harder you pull at that elastic band—and the more aggressive those measures are going to be, snapping you back. "It's not fair," you might be thinking—and you're right. It's *not* fair. But, as my dad has been known to say, "Who are you going to e-mail about it?"

Of course, genes don't *cause* obesity; they simply set you up for it. Many of my patients have siblings or close relatives who aren't overweight or obese. It takes environment to close the loop. The reality is that it's something you're *doing* that triggers those genes.

The example I always give to illustrate the nature-nurture interaction is skin cancer. You can walk around with the gene for skin cancer your whole life without anything bad happening to you. It's only when that gene for melanoma is "turned on" by exposure to the sun that the cancer actually develops.

The same thing is true about obesity. You may have a genetic propensity toward weight gain. But you have to do something to turn that genetic propensity on—and in this case, it's a propensity you turn on with food and a lack of physical activity.

Given the health risks associated with obesity, why in the world would our bodies set us up to fail in this way? Well, the short answer is: That's not really the way our bodies see it. In fact, they think they're setting us up for survival.

Let me explain. During the time when the great majority of our genetic material was established, the real threat to human health wasn't excess food and obesity but the exact opposite. A steady supply of food was by no means guaranteed for our hunter-gatherer ancestors, and starvation was a real threat. So the people who were best able to take advantage of the abundant times by storing energy as fat were more likely to survive when times were tight and there wasn't a woolly mammoth dinner in sight.

**The bodies of our hunter-gatherer ancestors evolved
to hoard calories and store fat;
their ability to do so was a survival advantage.**

Scientists call this the thrifty gene hypothesis. But times of plenty were short-lived for our ancestors, which is why they didn't suffer any of the consequences of being overweight.

The problem, of course, is that in twenty-first-century America, we have access to far too *many* calories, as opposed to too few. You don't have to look much further than a commercial strip in any town to see the problem. Our roads are literally lined with high-calorie, highly processed foods; at any fast-food chain in the country, you can eat a day's worth of calories and a week's worth of saturated fat in ten minutes, and for just five or six dollars.

**It has never been so easy—
or so cheap—
to consume so many calories.**

Add to that some other fundamental changes in our food habits and lifestyle habits, and you have what amounts to a real disaster. Drs. Lisa Young and Marion Nestle published a study in the *American Journal of Public Health* in 2002 in which they compared commonly available food servings with the recommended portions of those foods. Their findings were chilling; we regularly eat *many times* what we should. To give some examples: The cookies they looked at were as much as seven times standard portion sizes; servings of pasta were often as much as five times standard portion size; muffins weighed three times what they should. And in one of the most commonly cited findings of this study, they noted that in the 1950s, McDonald's only offered one size of fries—a small—which weighed a third of what the largest size weighed in 2001.

Not only do we have access to *more* food than ever before, but for the most part, it's *worse* food. The highly processed, sugar-laden nature of the food available at fast-food restaurants packs a much bigger caloric punch than whatever most of our great-grandparents ate at home. They didn't have packaged chips and snack cakes loaded with twenty unpronounceable ingredients available at every gas station and corner deli. Disturbing evidence shows that Americans get a large proportion of their calories from sugary liquids, such as sodas and sports drinks, which have no nutritional value at all. Check the side of the bottle: Even most commonly available juices are made with only a small percentage of actual fruit juice—and more sugar (or high-fructose corn syrup) than is healthy for anyone.

Highly processed foods, including sugary sodas and refined grains, also tend to mess with your blood sugar. When you eat what we call high-glycemic foods, sugars are released very rapidly into your bloodstream. Your blood sugar goes way up, and your body dumps a lot of insulin into your system to compensate. Not only does this process feel bad (you feel speedy and sick when your blood sugar spikes, and spent when it crashes)—but as soon as your blood sugar comes down, you're hungry again. So you eat again, and get hungry again, and the numbers on the scale inch ever higher.

The other big change that's taken place over the last few generations is that we're really not burning any of those extra calories off over the course of our day. I laughed out loud when I heard comedian Ellen DeGeneres say that Americans are too lazy even to chew gum; we need breath strips, which melt in our mouths without any effort from us at all. Jokes aside, there has been a steady and dramatic decrease in physical activity, and we're seeing the results in our waistlines. Your grandmother didn't go through a drive-in window, and she didn't eat in her car. She carried her groceries *home* (not just to the trunk), and just doing the family's laundry would have constituted a serious workout. Now, I'm not suggesting that we get rid of our washer-driers, but we do have to replace that lost movement somehow. Our bodies are healthiest when we move, on a regular basis—and yet, on an average day, the majority of us move very little: from our parking space to our desks, back to the car eight hours later, through the drive-through, and then onto the couch.

Nobody suffers from this lack of activity more than our kids. When my dad was in elementary school, he not only had a daily gym class but also two recesses that took place on a playground; after school he played outside with his buddies until dark. I will have to work very hard to make sure that my daughter gets even a small percentage of that exercise, given the prevalence of television and video games and the way physical education has largely been phased out in schools.

Factors in our environment may have changed, but our genes have not. And *that's* how we have ended up with an obesity epidemic: Excess calories are everywhere we look, and our thrifty genes keep greedily socking those excess calories away in the form of fat—insurance against a famine that never comes. So it's not just nature *or* nurture, but a combination of the two.

Nature and nurture aren't the only factors, either. There's a strong psychological component to weight gain as well, and it's one that we ignore at our peril if we're looking for a permanent solution to obesity.

Let's face it—most of us don't just use food as fuel. It's a friend when we're feeling isolated, a distraction when we're bored, a mood elevator when we're feeling depressed, a security blanket when we're anxious, a numbing agent when we're feeling too much. It's a habit, too: We get used to sitting down in front of the television with a bag of chips when we come home after school, and years later, we find ourselves doing the same thing when we arrive home after work. Food is also a way to connect with the people around us; in many cultures, food is at the center of every gathering, and in many families, food is a way to give and get affection. Feeding *these* hungers can go well beyond what our bodies need to survive.

Becoming seriously overweight is often a response to a significant trauma as well. The correlation between obesity and sexual or physical abuse in childhood is astronomical; the extra weight creates a permanent, portable protective barrier between the obese person and a harmful outside world. A period of tremendous sadness may precipitate a weight gain: A number of my patients have told me that they gained their weight after the death of a parent or of a child. "I thought, 'If I can get through this, I deserve to eat anything I want,'" one told me. And so she did, medicating her tremendous pain with food.

Even tremendous happiness can get you into trouble: One of my patients came back to see me for help after he'd begun to gain back some of the weight he'd lost after his surgery. The reason? He'd fallen in love with a terrific woman, found a new job, and moved into his dream house—and amid all that happiness, his new and improved food habits had fallen to the bottom of the list of priorities.

So, no—it's not quite as simple as just putting the fork down.

**Genes, environmental influences, habits, and our
emotional relationship to food *all* contribute
to obesity.**

And the failure to address the multitude of factors contributing to this disease is why the majority of diets don't work.

So what does? What's the best solution to address the multiple factors causing obesity? Well, I believe that for many people, it's weight loss surgery—and the National Institutes of Health agrees. But we'll get there in a minute. First, let's look at the alternatives—and why I believe they've let so many people down.

Nonsurgical Weight-Loss Strategies

By the time most of my patients come to me, they've tried a number of strategies to lose weight, usually over many years. We're bombarded with them: the new, quick-results, no-fail diet featured in every magazine, the miracle supplements advertised on television and radio.

Here's why and how these strategies so often fail them over the long term:

Conventional Diets

> *"I do WeightWatchers every year, and lose about forty pounds. Then I put it back on, plus five or ten pounds. I've been doing this since my teens."*

Eighty percent of dieters are successful in losing weight. It's simple math: Eat fewer calories than you burn, and you will lose weight. There are lots of programs out there to help you do that.

But I'm sure I'm not telling you anything you don't know when I say that the weight loss often isn't permanent. People can take the weight off, but they can't keep it off, and when they gain it back, they usually gain it back with a little extra for their trouble. We talked about that genetically determined set point earlier, and that's what's at work here. Your body thinks it's starving, and when that rubber band snaps back, it does so with a vengeance. Your metabolism slows, you're hungrier, and the weight comes back—plus some. The cycle has been called lots of things, including yo-yo dieting, and it's how people diet their way all the way to morbid obesity.

What's usually prescribed for someone struggling with excess weight? A low calorie diet, usually between 1000 and 1200 calories. But studies show that traditionally these diets result in only a 5 to 8 percent loss of excess weight—that's a total of 8 pounds in someone who is 100 pounds overweight.

Why doesn't cutting calories work? Two main reasons: 1) People underestimate the number of calories they consume by about 50 percent—so that 1200 calorie diet is really probably closer to 1800 by the end of the day, and 2), people just get too hungry to stay on these diets. A hormone called ghrelin controls hunger. As you diet, your ghrelin level gets higher and higher, making you hungrier and hungrier. That's why when you start a diet, it's relatively easy to say no when you're offered a piece of cake. "No thanks, I'm dieting," you say—and it's really no hardship. A couple of weeks later, someone offers you that same piece of cake, and you can't stop thinking about it: "Is that Betty Crocker?" Eat that piece of cake, and you'll blame your willpower—but what you should blame is the ghrelin. It's making you hungrier than you were a few weeks ago.

So low-calorie diets don't work. Very-low-calorie diets, such as Optifast, Medifast, and HMR, which usually top out at 800 calories a day, are often very effective; study participants have been shown to lose between 15 and 25 percent of their excess weight at sixteen to eighteen weeks. But these diets come with a host of problems as well. Because they provide for less than 1000 calories a day, they must be done under close medical supervision: malnutrition, electrolyte imbalance, gallstone formation, and dehydration are often side effects. And while initial weight loss is very good, compliance is absolutely terrible: If people have a hard time staying on the so-called low-calorie diets, when they're eating between 1200 and 1800 calories, you can only imagine how they respond when their allowed calories are cut in half again. So long-term weight loss with these programs is very poor.

Low- and very-low-calorie diets aren't the only diets out there, of course, as a walk through the diet book section at your local bookstore will quickly show. But none of them work much better as a solution for obesity. A study in the *Journal of the American Medical Association* looked at a number of the most popular over-the-counter diets, including Atkins, the Zone, Ornish, and LEARN. Atkins was the best of the lot—but total weight loss in overweight and obese women was only ten pounds over the course of a year. That's just not enough to make a significant difference for the majority of my patients.

I'm not saying that conventional diets are completely ineffective. If you're twenty, thirty, even fifty pounds overweight, I can think of no better solution than a reduced-calorie diet of high-quality, unrefined foods and a regular exercise program. But I do think—and both the anecdotal evidence and the science back me up—that conventional diets are ineffective treatments *for obesity.*

Exercise

"I looked at one of those charts online that tells you how many calories you've burned for the different activities. I'd worked out for an hour, and I hadn't even made a dent in my breakfast."

Exercise is widely heralded as an effective strategy for weight loss. But is it an effective treatment for the obese?

Not really. I hesitate to say a single bad word about exercise because it is so vital to health. In fact, there are many studies that show that you can in fact be "fit and fat"—something that is far better than fat and sedentary. We'll talk about the benefits of exercise—and there are a lot of them—in Chapter 14. But if you're obese and exercising for weight loss, I have to be honest: The math doesn't look good.

Let me explain. Let's say you decide that you want to lose 100 pounds over the course of a year. To lose one pound, you must have a net calorie deficit of 3800 calories. So to lose 100 pounds, you would have to eat 380,000 calories less than you burn. Over the year, that means burning about 1000 calories a day over what you're eating. (The average overweight individual is taking in about 3500 calories a day and burning about 1700. So you are 1800 calories positive, or 2800 calories above your goal.)

But 1000 calories is a lot of calories to cut out of your usual diet, and as we discussed earlier in the chapter, your body isn't going to make this easy to do. You're going to feel some real hunger pangs in the process. So maybe you think you'll just burn more calories with exercise. The problem is that strenuous exercise—not a walk in the park but a real sweaty session—only burns about 10 calories per minute. So, even if you cut your diet by 1000 calories a day, you still would have to work out three hours a day to lose that 100 pounds in a year. *Three hours a day!* (In case you were wondering, this is how the contestants on shows like *The Biggest Loser* shed those pounds through diet and exercise. Not only are they on low-calorie diets, but they work out for hours every day.)

Now, I love exercise, but I couldn't do it for three hours a day, every day, and I doubt you have the time or means to do it, either. That's not to say you shouldn't exercise—in fact, exercise is as essential to your long-term success as anything else. But exercise as a realistic weight-loss solution for the obese? The math just doesn't work.

Pharmaceutical Approaches

> *"Yeah, I lost weight on the drugs. I just couldn't ever be more than ten feet away from a toilet."*

Trust me, folks: The search is out there for a magic pill. There's certainly a pot of gold at the end of that rainbow for the lucky researcher or pharmaceutical company that comes up with a medication to successfully address the weight problems that 70 percent of Americans deal with.

But they haven't found it yet, and in the rush to push something effective onto the market, there have been some pretty scary mistakes. Fen-phen increased metabolism and tricked the body into feeling less hungry; it also caused valvular heart disease. People got great results with rimonabant, a drug that blocks certain receptors in the brain (the same receptors that give marijuana smokers the munchies); unfortunately, they not only lost weight, but they also lost their will to live as well. The FDA ultimately rejected rimonabant in 2007 because of its strong links to depression.

That said, there are three drugs currently on the market that have been clinically proven to help people lose weight. (Bear in mind, however, that all are far from perfect.)

- **Orlistat** (Xenical, Alli), which works by blocking the body's ability to absorb fat. Many patients stop using these drugs, however, because they come with some unfortunate side effects. If the fat is not being absorbed, it's got to come out somewhere, and trust me, it isn't pretty.

- **Sibutramine** (Meridia), which works on several chemicals in the brain in much the same way as many of the antidepressant medications. The result is a reduction in hunger.

- **Phentermine** (Adipex), which stimulates the central nervous system to make you less hungry.

Although these drugs do produce results, there have been concerns about safety issues with them. And sibutramine and phentermine increase blood pressure, something that's already a problem for most obese people. Additionally, phentermine is considered to be habit forming, and so it is only approved for twelve weeks of use—hardly a sound approach to what should be a lifetime journey.

The safety issues with these drugs are a concern, but the cost-benefit ratio might work—if only they were more effective. A review of eleven orlistat studies and five sibutramine studies found that both medications combined with a weight-loss diet resulted in weight loss of less than five kilograms (eleven pounds), as compared to a placebo. Eleven pounds! That's great if you're a normal-weight person who has picked up a couple of pounds after the holidays, but it's just not significant enough to affect the obesity epidemic. In another study, at three years out on orlistat, participants had lost just 8 to 10 percent of excess weight, and only eight pounds more than people taking the placebo. And there is no good science on long-term weight loss with phentermine at all.

The search for a weight-loss pill will continue. But I think we can agree that the solutions currently available are not viable ones for the obese.

⦚⦚⦚⦚⦚⦚⦚⦚

In the previous chapter, we talked about the costs of obesity. There is also a cost to these ineffective strategies: the disappointment of family and friends, the disapproval of your doctor, and a feeling of personal failure all eventually give way to depression, anxiety, low self-esteem, and an unhealthy preoccupation with food.

**Diet and drug strategies don't just fail the obese;
they make the obese feel like they have failed.**

Understanding how seriously this disease affects people's health and lives makes the search for an effective solution even more imperative. In this chapter, we talked about the complex group of factors that contribute to this disease. It's time now to look at the best solution to this problem that we currently have—and how to determine whether it's the right solution for you.

CHAPTER THREE

Weight-Loss Surgery

A Real Solution

"My bypass changed my life. My only regret is that I didn't have it done ten years ago."

"Surgery is the hardest thing I've ever done; it was also the best."

"I thought it was me. But I now know that I can exercise, eat healthily, and maintain a normal weight—as long as my body's not fighting me the whole way."

If you've seen *Big Medicine*, you know that I often tease my dad about being "old-school." But for all my talk, I'm consistently impressed by the way he keeps up with the most cutting-edge research and the newest procedures. So I guess it shouldn't have been a tremendous surprise that he was the one who started doing weight-loss surgery first.

I should first tell you that my dad is unquestionably the reason I am a surgeon today. I used to do rounds with him at the hospital when other kids were playing baseball with their dads. This is probably why I'm no good at baseball, but I do think that my early exposure to such a great role model made me a pretty good doctor.

And yet, as much as I trust my father's judgment, I was a little hesitant to follow in his footsteps with weight-loss surgery. Looking back on it now, I realize that my hesitance was born out of misinformation. First of all, I confess that—like many other medical professionals—I thought that obesity was the patient's fault. I've always been a fairly health-conscious person, someone who found it relatively easy to maintain a normal weight and who enjoyed exercise, and I thought, "If I can do it, why can't these people?" Weight-loss surgery seemed to me like an overaggressive solution to what I thought was essentially a cosmetic problem. To make matters worse, I had been led by the doctors who trained me to believe that these surgeries were loaded with complications, and therefore they were very dangerous for the patient. Obviously, I had a lot of learning to do.

Reluctantly, but out of respect for my father, I took several weight-loss surgery courses, went to national meetings of the American Society for Metabolic and Bariatric Surgery, and visited a number of physicians who performed weight-loss surgery. I read books and journals about obesity and weight-loss surgery.

And I was completely shocked by what I learned. The research really turned my head. I hadn't realized the overwhelming evidence that obesity is a disease, and often an inherited one. I had absolutely no idea that conventional diets failed the obese at the rate that they do. So I studied the science of hunger and learned that there are hormones—such as ghrelin—that make certain people hungrier and predispose them toward having a slower metabolic rate. I was also startled to find that there is an absolute mountain of science showing that obesity surgery not only helps people lose weight but *cures disease*, and helps people live longer and more fulfilling lives.

But I still wasn't completely convinced. In fact, even after I'd started doing the surgeries, there were some doubts knocking around in my head. It wasn't until I started to see my postsurgical patients—and the unbelievable physical and medical transformations that are the daily stuff of a bariatric surgeon's practice—that I really dove in.

That was seven years ago, and I haven't looked back. Our practice is now pretty much exclusively weight-loss surgery. My sister is even a weight-loss surgery patient (not ours!). As far as I'm concerned, it is a gift to be able to make the kind of difference that I can now facilitate in my patients' lives. It's very common for my presurgical patients to describe feeling trapped in their bodies; they tell me that the surgery feels like the key they'd been searching for their whole lives. And when they throw open that door, their whole lives change.

Look Better, *Feel* Better

From a physician's perspective, the physical transformation we see after surgery is absolutely astonishing. Without hunger (or at least a significant reduction in it), the weight comes off. I've seen it hundreds of times, and still there is no describing the shock and pleasure I get from seeing someone lose a significant percentage of their excess weight. "One hundred and thirty pounds!" a patient said to me this morning. *"I've never weighed one hundred and thirty pounds as an adult."* I know lots of different kinds of surgeons; how many of their patients get up and twirl when they're called from the waiting room?

The cosmetic changes are significant, but the medical ones are even more impressive. One of the first things I do when I meet a new patient is ask them what medications they take. The answer, now familiar, saddens me every time. Most of my patients—even the young people—are taking pills by the handful to cope with diseases caused by obesity. Many of them bring a printed list so they won't forget any of them; one of them told me that she had once measured out a day's worth of pills and filled a large dinner plate with the result.

One of the most gratifying parts of my job, then, is revisiting that medication issue after surgery. As the pounds drop off, so do my patients' need for medications—often disappearing altogether.

**WLS patients feel better because they *are* better—
in a scientifically measurable way.**

As someone who has treated literally thousands of people, I can say without question that this surgery has the potential to alleviate or *cure* many obesity-related co-morbidities, including diabetes, high blood pressure, arthritis, asthma, reflux, sleep apnea, and a host of others.

In fact, this surgery is the *only* cure for many of these things. The results can be quite dramatic. Let me show you what I mean. A meta-analysis—a study that looks at the results of lots of other studies—of bariatric surgery was published in the *Journal of the American Medical Association* in 2004. Here's what they found:

Weight loss. On average, was 61.2 percent of excess weight. Patients who had the band lost 47.5 percent of their excess weight; patients who had the bypass lost 61.6 percent of their excess weight. People who had the biliopancreatic diversion or duodenal switch lost 70.1 percent of their excess weight. (Don't worry; we'll go into the differences between all of these surgeries a little later in the chapter.)

Very impressive, as I'm sure you'll agree. But here's what really knocked my socks off:

Diabetes was completely resolved in 76.8 percent of patients and resolved or improved in 86.0 percent. There have been more than thirty studies confirming this result—some with even more dramatic findings.

Hyperlipidemia (elevated cholesterol levels) were improved in 70 percent or more of patients.

Hypertension was resolved in 61.7 percent of patients and resolved or improved in 78.5 percent.

Obstructive sleep apnea was resolved in 85.7 percent of patients and was resolved or improved in 83.6 percent of patients.

High cholesterol was reduced in more than 70 percent of patients.

GERD was 72 to 98 percent resolved.

And, according to the American Society for Metabolic and Bariatric Surgery's Web site:

Asthma was 82 percent improved or resolved.

Cardiovascular disease showed a 82 percent risk reduction of heart attack or stroke. One study showed that this surgery was more effective at preventing heart attacks than angioplasty was.

Degenerative joint disease was 41 to 76 percent resolved.

Depression was 55 percent resolved.

Gout was 77 percent resolved.

Metabolic syndrome was 80 percent resolved.

Nonalcoholic fatty liver disease was 90 percent improved for steatosis; there was a 37 percent resolution of inflammation and 20 percent resolution of fibrosis.

Pseudotumors were 95 percent resolved.

PCOS (Polycystic Ovarian Syndrome) was 79 percent resolved for hirsutism and there was a 100 percent resolution of menstrual irregularities.

Venous stasis disease was 95 percent resolved.

Those numbers are deeply, deeply significant. "Resolved" means *cured*. To put it into perspective, if a drug company announced a new pharmaceutical with the ability to resolve this many diseases at this impressive a rate, it would be a blockbuster. Nothing currently on the market even compares. Diabetic medications may help control blood sugar, but they do not cure diabetes. Statin drugs only help with cholesterol when you're taking them. Arthritis medications simply mask the pain; they don't unload the joints, which is what fixes them. And none of these drugs work for everyone. In fact, they're usually less effective in the obese; for instance, diabetics get more and more resistant to their medications the heavier they get.

And yet here is a surgery that can singlehandedly wipe out some of the most insidious co-morbidities associated with obesity.

In truth, the numbers above can get even better, depending on which surgery you choose. Gastric bypass, for example, is such an effective treatment for diabetes that there recently was a conference in Rome dedicated to looking at whether this might be a viable surgery *for diabetics who aren't obese.* The conclusion was that it may very well be—and further studies are being done.

A study published in the January 2008 issue of the *Journal of the American Medical Association* put this question to bed. "Weight-loss surgery works much better than standard medical therapy as a treatment for Type 2 diabetes in obese people," trumpeted the front-page story in the *New York Times*. The studies led the society of bariatric surgeons—formerly known as the American Society for Bariatric Surgeons—to change its name to the American Society for Metabolic and Bariatric Surgery in response. In other words, we don't just treat weight with this surgery; we also treat metabolic disorders such as diabetes.

As satisfying as the results of that meta-analysis might have been, I can also tell you that the list of conditions resolved or improved by these surgeries is nowhere near comprehensive. Every day someone walks into my office and tells me that some health problem they didn't even know was related to their obesity—erectile dysfunction, skin rashes, chronic fatigue—has resolved since they lost their weight.

But here's my favorite study result of all:

Quality of life was improved in 95 percent of patients.

It's not a surprise: I don't know any genuinely happy, healthy people who hate their bodies—do you?

After surgery, my patients can cross their legs. They can tie their shoelaces—they can see their shoes! They can set a computer on their laps. They can go to the movies and the theater, and they travel more comfortably on airplanes. They can sit in a booth at a restaurant, ride roller coasters, and keep up with their kids. They often gain the confidence, energy, and health to tackle challenges and pursue long-held dreams.

Some bariatric patients refer to the date of their surgery as "their second birthday," because that's how they see it—as a rebirth. While an improvement in quality of life may not be quantifiable, I believe that it alone has a big impact on my patients' overall health.

CHAPTER FOUR

The Nuts and Bolts of Weight-Loss Surgery

We've reviewed a number of pretty convincing arguments for weight-loss surgery. But what do these surgeries actually entail?

There are a number of different types of weight-loss surgeries. But before we talk about the specific surgeries, it's important to have a basic understanding of the parts in question. A brief anatomy lesson:

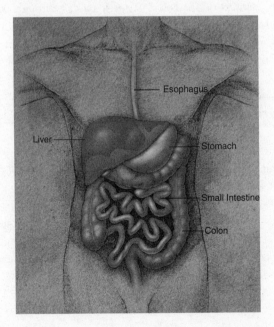

You eat food. When you swallow, the food travels from the mouth into the esophagus—a long, muscular tube connecting the mouth to the stomach. At the base of the esophagus, where the esophagus and stomach connect, is a sphincter, or a band of muscle that tightens and prevents food from coming back up. The stomach itself is a relatively large, stretchable pouch, that can hold about 2000 cc, approximately the contents of a two-liter soda bottle. There the food mixes with hydrochloric acid and a number of other digestive juices to break the food down.

From the stomach, food passes through another sphincter called the pyloric valve into the small intestine, which is between fifteen and twenty feet long. The first section of the small intestine is called the duodenum; this is where the partially digested food is mixed with bile from the liver and juices from the pancreas. Iron and calcium are absorbed here.

Next, food passes into the middle section, which is known as the jejunum, and, finally, into the last section of the small intestine, called the ileum. These two sections are where the majority of calories and vitamins are taken out of the food stream and converted into forms the body can use.

From the small intestine, food travels through yet another sphincter into the large intestine, or colon. After it passes through the colon, it's eliminated from the body as waste. Food—and therefore calories—is absorbed all throughout the small intestine but not in the colon.

A NOTE ABOUT RISK
"Is weight-loss surgery dangerous?"

This is a question I hear a lot when I tell people what I do, largely because of the way these surgeries used to be done and because of the way they've been portrayed in the media.

All major surgery carries serious risks, and this one is no exception. I will go through those risks very closely and carefully with you—just as I do with my patients—in the chapters that follow. But before I do, I'd like to say one thing, which is that:

**If you are morbidly obese,
you are more likely to die *without* the surgery
than you are *from* it.**

An excellent study in Canada followed two groups of obese patients: one group who had WLS surgery; one who didn't. Patients were followed for several years, and the researchers saw something surprising: The people who had had the surgery had an *89 percent* reduced risk of death during that period compared to those who didn't. The authors of the study concluded that weight-loss surgery significantly decreases overall mortality as well as the development of new health-related conditions.

How Weight-Loss Surgery Works

When we talk about weight-loss surgery, it's not a single surgery we're talking about but a number of different procedures (the band, for example, or the bypass) that use a variety of means to achieve the same end: helping you lose a significant amount of weight. Part of the decision to have these surgeries is determining—in concert with your doctors—which one is right for you. (More on figuring this out in Chapter 5.)

There are three different ways that weight-loss surgery can help you to lose weight.

Restrictive. Surgeries in this category simply reduce the amount of food the stomach can hold by reducing the size of the stomach.

Malabsorptive. Surgeries in this category change the architecture of the digestive tract, limiting the number of calories and nutrients that the body can absorb from food.

Combination. This third category is a combination of the two previous ones.

A Brief History of Weight-Loss Surgery

There are a lot of misconceptions about weight-loss surgery, and many of them stem from the various ways these procedures were done in the past. So I'd like to begin this section with a brief history—and how those earlier attempts compare to the procedures done today.

The first surgery for weight loss was done in the 1950s. The surgeons at that time reasoned that cutting the small intestines short could create a situation whereby some food—and therefore some calories—would not be absorbed. The surgery was called the jejunal-ileal or JI bypass. If you know someone who had a bypass in the 70s, this surgery is what they had.

The theory proved correct. Patients could eat whatever they wanted and still lose weight because their bodies failed to absorb all the calories. But if you don't absorb food, it comes out the other end. Patients had terrible diarrhea after this surgery—and they also suffered from serious nutrient deficiencies because they were not absorbing important vitamins.

The JI bypass was largely abandoned, and the next phase in weight-loss surgery was a shift away from "malabsorption" surgeries to a more restrictive type, one that didn't allow the patient to eat very much. Surgeons tried many different ways of stapling or banding the stomach to separate out a smaller portion of the stomach. Dr. Edward Mason, who is one of the fathers of weight-loss surgery, developed a procedure called the vertical banded gastroplasty (VBG). He stapled the stomach in a vertical line, partitioning it so that the top of the stomach formed a type of chamber. At the base of that chamber, Dr. Mason placed a plastic band, that helped delay the passage of food and led to a feeling of fullness. If you know someone who had their stomach stapled or banded in the 1980s, this is what they had.

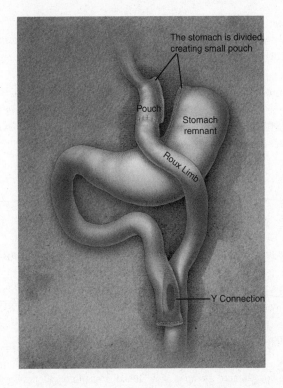

The VBG surgery worked for a while, but, unfortunately, people would often gain the weight back because the surgically created chamber would dilate, the staples would break down, and the partition would disappear. There was also frequent vomiting because the band used in those days was one-size-fits-all, and sometimes it was too tight; if food can't get through, it comes back up. But their loss was our gain: The success and failures of these early experiments lead to an unbelievable amount of research into just about every detail of weight-loss surgery that you could possibly imagine—and to the highly effective options that exist today.

We'll now take a close look at the most commonly performed and accepted surgeries used now. In this section, I'll not only explain how the surgeries work and what they entail, but I'll also outline what I consider the major risks and benefits of each to be. I usually have an opinion about which surgery is best for a given patient, and your surgeon will as well. But as I always tell my patients, the decision is really in their hands; my responsibility is to make sure they have the information they need to make it.

Please note: Unlike the procedures described above, the surgeries below are *not* experimental. They all come with an amazing amount of research into their efficacy and safety—and they have helped to genuinely transform the lives of tens of thousands of people.

OPEN OR CLOSED?

All of the procedures discussed below can be done one of two ways: open or laparoscopically.

Open surgery, which is the way these surgeries were all done once upon a time, means that the surgeon has to make a very large incision in the abdomen. This not only means a longer recovery period, but it also increases risk for infection and problems with wound healing (often an issue with the obese).

Advances in surgery now allow these procedures to be done *laparoscopically*. In a laparoscopic procedure, the surgeon makes five or six very small incisions along the abdomen, just big enough for the surgical instruments to be passed through—including a small camera that projects an image onto a screen. The surgeon performs the operation using this image to guide him instead of looking into the actual abdominal cavity.

Why do some surgeons perform these surgeries open? Laparoscopy requires that the surgeon be trained in comparatively newer techniques, and the hospital must also have the new equipment. There are many very good bariatric surgeons who do a fantastic job with open surgery—they might even argue that they do a *better* job than their colleagues who choose laparoscopy. And while I would never discourage anyone from going to one of these excellent surgeons, I personally believe that times have advanced, and that weight-loss surgeries are best performed through smaller incisions. The hospital stay is shorter and the rate of infection is greatly reduced. Also, the scars are much smaller—a cosmetic consideration, but also a medical one—in the event you need more abdominal surgery in the future, scar tissue can be difficult to work around.

In very rare cases—a lot of scar tissue, an anatomical anomaly, or in the case of a revision of a previous surgery, which can be more complicated—I will do these procedures open. But in my opinion, the majority of cases should be done laparoscopically.

Gastric Bypass

The most commonly performed weight-loss surgery in the United States is the gastric bypass. It's also called the Roux-en-Y, after the French doctor Roux who first did it, pronounced *Roo-en-why*. You may have seen it abbreviated as RNY; I will call it the bypass, or the gastric bypass, throughout this book.

The procedure. As mentioned, the stomach can hold up to 2000 cc. During gastric bypass surgery, we pass a balloon into the stomach, which can hold about 20 cc. We then use special surgical staplers to cut and divide the stomach around this tube; this creates a small, new stomach, which is often referred to as a "pouch," at the end of the esophagus.

Next, we go down to the small intestine—to the jejunum—and divide the intestine. We bring the distal (or farthest) part of the intestine—which is called the Roux limb—up to the pouch, and connect the two with staples or stitches. This connection is called an anastomosis. We finish up by taking the rest of the intestine and joining it up with the bottom of the Roux limb.

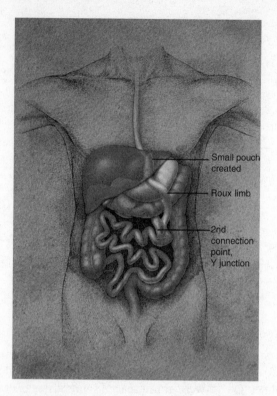

Small pouch created

Roux limb

2nd connection point, Y junction

Many people ask me what happens with the "old" stomach. It still functions and makes acids and digestive juices, which flow into the duodenum, where it joins juices from the liver and pancreas. This mixture of digestive juices goes from the duodenum into the jejunum, where it meets up with the food at the Y junction (hence the name of the surgery). Here it combines with the food, allowing it to be digested and absorbed as it makes its way through the rest of the small intestine. It's here that the majority of the nutrients and calories are absorbed.

How it works. The gastric bypass is in the third category described above, meaning that it is both restrictive and malabsorptive. That said, it is mainly a restrictive procedure—it works because it limits what you can eat. The pouch that we create in the stomach holds much less than what the ordinary stomach can hold, so you get full on less food. Generally, in the beginning it's difficult to get more than 1 to 2 ounces into your new pouch. The stomach does stretch, though; by six months and after, the average bypass patient consumes about 4 to 6 ounces at a sitting and a total of about 1200 calories a day.

But there is a malabsorptive component to the bypass as well, meaning not every calorie you eat is absorbed. When the food leaves the pouch and hits the Roux limb, it hasn't yet been mixed with the mixture of digestive juices, so it travels down the Roux limb but isn't digested until it hits the jejunum at the Y junction, which results in fewer calories and nutrients absorbed. Many more calories and nutrients are absorbed with this surgery than with the original JI bypass, however, or with the duodenal switch, which we will discuss later. So bypass patients do not typically have diarrhea, and they usually do not develop deficiencies—provided they take their vitamins and supplements!

HOW LONG IS MY ROUX LIMB?
The Distal Versus Proximal Debate

The amount of malabsorption a patient experiences after a gastric bypass depends on the length of the Roux limb. In WLS Web chat rooms, you may hear people talking about proximal and distal bypasses. In general, most bypasses are proximal, meaning that the Roux limb is fairly short. The distal bypass creates more malabsorption, and more problems as a result. Many people believe that a long, or distal, Roux limb is better for the severely obese because the calories go further without being absorbed. This may result in better weight loss, but it may also create more complications, given vitamin and protein deficiencies.

The bypass is a successful weight-loss tool for a few other reasons as well. First of all, one of the parts of the stomach that is bypassed when the pouch is created is the part that produces the hormone ghrelin, which stimulates appetite. The less ghrelin you have, the less hungry you are—and bypass patients have *much* less ghrelin; in fact, one study showed that bypass patients had 70 percent less ghrelin in their blood than people who were just dieting. So the bypass really can free you from being constantly driven by hunger and cravings; those messages simply aren't being sent to your brain.

The other way that the bypass helps you lose weight is, oddly enough, through an unpleasant side effect called dumping syndrome. We'll talk about dumping syndrome in more detail in Chapter 10, but, simply put: After the bypass, sugars and very refined carbohydrates can make you sick. Since sugars are one of the big things you want to avoid when you're trying to lose weight—and since getting ill is usually a very effective deterrent—the fact that you "dump" after a bypass reduces the likelihood that you'll use high-calorie soft foods such as ice cream to sabotage your tiny pouch. (It's not torture: Most people lose their taste for sweets after the surgery.)

Dumping happens in about 80 percent of patients—and those that don't dump wish they did because it makes it so much easier to say no to sugar.

What you can expect. On average, after gastric bypass surgery, patients lose about 60 to 75 percent of their excess weight. So let's say you're 100 pounds overweight; with the bypass, you can expect to lose about 60 to 75 pounds. If you're highly motivated in the diet and exercise department, you can lose even more. (Bear in mind that the opposite is also true: If you're not sufficiently committed to exercise and to eating more healthfully, you may lose less.)

The long-term data on these surgeries is very good. A recent study reviewed the excess weight loss fifteen years after gastric bypass, and found that, on average, people kept over 50 percent of their excess weight off. We do the surgery differently (and better) now, and are seeing even better weight loss as a result. What we typically see is patients losing 80 to 85 percent of their excess weight, gaining a bit back, and leveling off at about 60 to 70 percent of excess weight. I recently reviewed my database and found that the average weight loss in my patients one year after surgery was 73 percent; two years out, it was 70 percent.

You can also expect to see a significant reduction in the co-morbidities of obesity with this procedure. The big one here is diabetes. As we've discussed, the gastric bypass is a stunningly effective cure for type 2 diabetes; up to 96 percent of patients see a cure or an improvement. It's often instantaneous—I generally send diabetic patients home from the hospital without their meds—and very effective, even for people whose disease has been severe or very difficult to manage with medications.

As the weight comes off, we see a resolution in other morbidities, including high blood pressure, sleep apnea, GERD, and arthritis pain, as well.

Risks

While there are risks associated with the gastric bypass, I'm happy to report that they're nowhere near as dire as the media has made them sound; in fact, they're really quite low.

Some of them are also somewhat patient-dependent, which means that there are things you can do—like losing as much weight as you can before the surgery, not indulging in tons of high-fat foods in the weeks leading up to surgery, and exercising as soon as you possibly can and as much as you possibly can afterward—that affect your level of risk. (As you'll see in Chapter 6, the experience level of your surgeon is also a major factor.)

People are always worried about dying during or after surgery. In truth, this is a very rare occurrence. I have never lost a patient, and most big studies show a mortality rate of less than 0.3 percent. What that means is that you have more risk of dying while getting your heart operated on or your knee replaced.

BETTER AND BETTER

The risk profile for weight-loss surgery continues to drop drastically across the board.

A study done by the Agency for Healthcare Research and Quality (AHRQ) showed that the mortality rate associated with all types of bariatric surgery had dropped precipitously—by 78.7 percent!—from 0.89 percent in 1998 to 0.19 percent in 2004.

Here are the complications we see with the bypass:

Leaks. The biggest risk is that the connection between the new stomach pouch and the bowel can leak. This is a serious complication: Intestinal contents can leak into the abdomen, causing infection and abscess. As long as the leak is caught early, it can be repaired. I have greatly reduced incidences of leaks in my practice by checking the connection a number of ways before I complete the surgery. I insert a scope through the mouth while the patient is still asleep, look directly at the connection and blow air into it. I also use a dye to check for a leak. That way I can be certain before the patient even leaves the operating room that the connection is intact.

Leaks can still occur, and they do in 0.5 to 5 percent of cases. Symptoms of a leak include high heart rate, fever, or severe postsurgical pain (above and beyond what we normally expect to see). Leaks are diagnosed by having the patient swallow a dye or by taking a CAT scan.

Most leaks can be treated simply by resting the stomach, which means taking food through an IV for a while. Sometimes surgery needs to be done; we can also place a plastic stent in the pouch, through the mouth, to cover the leak. And if a leak results in an abscess, the abscess often can be drained by a radiologist, who will use a CAT scan to guide a small drain into the abscess.

Blood clots. Blood clots are always a risk with surgery, and people who are overweight have an increased tendency to get them, especially during surgery.

We are usually able to avoid clots by using blood thinners after (and sometimes before) surgery, as well as special boots with balloons that periodically inflate and squeeze the lower legs to keep the blood flowing. Another very effective strategy is to get the patient up and walking immediately. Keeping active after surgery is your best defense.

We suspect blood clots if the leg becomes swollen or painful, and we confirm the diagnosis by doing an ultrasound of the blood vessels of the leg. If a clot is found, your doctor will give you a blood thinner, sometimes for months after surgery. The real danger with clots is that they can break off and travel to the lung. This is called pulmonary embolism, and it is very dangerous; fortunately, it seldom occurs.

If you have had a blood clot, or even a family history of clotting disorders, tell your surgeon. He or she may want to put a special filter into the main vein leaving your leg, which will catch a clot before it gets to your lungs. (This is an outpatient procedure, done before surgery in high-risk patients.)

Bowel obstruction. During the bypass, We reroute the intestines: We cut and reconnect them to the Roux limb. As a result, it is possible to develop a twist in the intestine, also called an internal hernia; unfortunately, this can happen anytime—even years out. We see this in about 3 to 5 percent of patients.

Patients know it's happening because they experience abdominal pain or swelling and vomiting. A CAT scan will confirm the diagnosis. Often surgery is required, but not always.

Ulcers. The pouch is very sensitive, and there is a risk of ulcer as a result. This risk is largely determined by patient behavior. For instance, I feel very confident saying that if you smoke after your surgery, you will get an ulcer. And you'll have to say good-bye to the class of drugs called NSAIDs, including Motrin, Aleve, Advil, Celebrex, and so on. (You'll find more information and a full list of off-limits drugs on page 137.) You can still take Tylenol and other pain-relieving medications, however, as approved by your surgeon.

The risk of ulcer is about 5 percent, although it may be more (I personally believe it's underreported), and it can happen even if you avoid NSAIDs and cigarettes. Ulcers present as burning pain; we confirm the diagnosis with an endoscopy, a scope down the esophagus. Ulcers can be treated with antacid medications; they very seldom require surgery.

Stricture. If there's a big buildup of scar tissue where we've attached your intestine to the pouch, it can narrow the opening, making it very difficult for food to enter. As a result, the patient vomits whenever he or she eats.

This happens in 5 to 8 percent of cases. When it does, we insert a scope into the pouch and inflate a balloon across the connection to the intestine. Blowing the balloon up breaks the scar tissue; rarely is surgery needed.

Bleeding. There is a risk of internal bleeding after a bypass—after all, we are cutting and dividing the intestines along with their blood supply and then giving the patient blood thinners—but the risk is very low. I would say that only about 1 percent of patients ever need a transfusion.

Wound infection. This happens much more commonly in open surgery, although it can also happen in the smaller, laparoscopic incisions. It is usually very minor and treated with antibiotics. On occasion we may have to open up the small wound and do daily dressing changes. I know this sounds awful, but opening the wound allows the infection to be cleaned out, and the wound then closes quickly.

Hernias. Hernia, an opening or weakness in the abdominal wall, also happens much more often with open surgery, although again, it does occur on rare occasions with laparoscopic incisions. This usually occurs months after surgery, and it is diagnosed when there is a bulging at the incision.

Nutritional deficiency. The bypass can result in several different vitamin deficiencies. The most common are B_{12}, calcium, vitamin D, iron, and thiamine. Deficiencies can show up as anemia, osteoporosis, and fatigue.

Fortunately, taking appropriate vitamins and supplements, as we will discuss later at greater length, will prevent these problems. I also advise patients to get their labs checked six months postoperatively, and then yearly afterward, to check for any deficiencies.

Nausea. Some people can be very nauseated after surgery. This usually gets better with time, and there are meds that can help until it passes.

Other. Other complications do occur, but *very rarely*. Lightning strikes, and so does stuff happen in surgery, but problems other than the ones we've discussed are extremely rare.

I believe that gastric bypass performed by a qualified surgeon is a safe procedure, and I'm happy to say that we've had very few complications in our practice.

IS IT REVERSIBLE?

People often ask me if the bypass is reversible. The answer is yes, but it is very difficult to do. And in my experience, no one ever asks once they've had the procedure.

I prefer that my patients be very sure that they want the bypass, and that they consider it irreversible.

ANOTHER NOTE ABOUT RISK

There are a few things to remember when you're talking about risks. The first is that the numbers cited in this chapter do vary—sometimes quite widely—from doctor to doctor. Some people are more proficient than others; some have had more practice; others go the extra step to reduce complications. That's why it's so important to have faith in your doctor—something we'll discuss in detail in Chapter 6.

The other issue, though, has to do with the finicky nature of statistics. Does your doctor have a higher mortality rate than another one because he takes on higher-risk patients? It might mean he's a really good surgeon and takes cases that other, less-experienced physicians wouldn't touch.

After all, the higher someone's BMI is, the more dangerous the surgery is. But the higher the BMI, the more risk a patient has of dying from obesity-related causes—which means that they need the intervention even more than their lighter-weight counterparts.

I don't think we want to create a world in which doctors are afraid to do what could be a life-saving operation on someone who's not an ideal candidate just because they don't want their statistics to suffer.

Gastric Band

The gastric band, or LAP-BAND device, was approved for use in the United States by the FDA in 2001, although it has been used in Europe since the 1990s.

The procedure. In this surgery—which is done laparoscopically (through several small incisions in the abdomen)—we encircle the upper stomach with a band and sew it in place. The band is made of silicone and Silastic. It has a balloon on its inner surface, which is connected to a tube, which leads to a small port (a small plastic connector about the size of a half-dollar) under the skin, on top of the muscle of the abdominal wall.

Through this port, your doctor will add or remove saline (salt water)

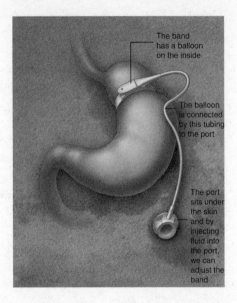

The band
has a balloon
on the inside

The balloon
is connected
by this tubing
to the port

The port
sits under
the skin
and by
injecting
fluid into
the port,
we can
adjust the
band

from the balloon during your follow-up visits, making it larger or smaller—and thus tighter or looser. (This is called a fill.)

How it works. The band is purely restrictive. When the band is made tighter, it decreases hunger by causing a stretching of the stomach above the band, which sends a message to your brain that you're full—even after a smaller portion of food. Unlike the bypass, the band does not create any changes in the hormones of the gut. There is also no malabsorption.

After the surgery you will need to visit your surgeon several times for fills. Your doctor can either make it tighter or looser if you're having difficulty getting food down.

What you can expect. Studies show that patients lose between 30 and 50 percent of their excess weight over three to five years. (In other words: If you're 100 pounds overweight, you can expect to lose between thirty and fifty pounds; in some studies, participants achieved up to 60 percent excess weight loss.) There are no results from long-term studies available in the United States yet, but the data from Europe and Australia shows that this weight may stay off long term.

Of course, that's true only *if the band stays on*. There are increasing reports from Europe of patients needing to have the band removed after several years because of slips or a failure to tolerate it. There is so much variability in the literature that I don't feel comfortable quoting a specific percentage of people who eventually need to have their bands removed, but it looks like it might be as high as 10 to 20 percent—certainly something that I'm keeping my eye on.

I also feel obliged to mention that while the weight loss in most studies is about 50 percent of excess weight, that is just an average; we see a lot of variability in our clinic. I do see patients who lose 80 percent, but I also see patients who lose only 20 percent. So that 50 percent is a true average.

Risks

As I tell my patients, the risks of serious complications are much fewer with the band than with the bypass, because there's no fundamental change in the anatomy. The risk of minor, annoying complications, however, is greater.

Band slip/erosion. As I mentioned above, the position of the band can slip, or it can erode into the stomach (more on this below), requiring another operation to fix it.

The stomach is constantly moving, and that movement can make the band slip into the wrong location. This is reported to happen in up to 10 percent of cases, which is not a small number. If the band slips, you will start vomiting and have difficulty keeping even liquids down. You'll also experience reflux.

A band slip is confirmed by doing an X-ray while the patient drinks a dye solution. Often, if we pull the fluid out of the band, the band slips back into place. Sometimes the band has to be surgically repositioned or removed.

An erosion is when the band actually grows into the stomach. This is fairly uncommon; it happens in about 1 percent of cases. We suspect it when the patient develops a port site infection in the skin. (The port is the place where we inject fluid to fill the band.) It is confirmed by placing a scope through the mouth into the stomach; treatment is always permanent removal of the band.

Port flip. In some cases, the port on the muscle of the abdominal wall "flips," or turns over, making it hard for the surgeon to access it for fills. It's inconvenient, but not serious, and it requires a minor procedure to correct it.

Port or band infection. This is rare, but possible. It requires a course of antibiotics, and possibly the removal of the band.

Hiatal hernia. A hiatal hernia is basically a widening of the opening in the diaphragm through which the esophagus passes as it enters the stomach. (If you have a hernia before surgery, we can fix it while placing the band.) The band tightens at the upper part of the stomach, which can cause this upper part to bulge and push on the diaphragm, opening a hernia.

The problem with a hiatal hernia in band patients is that it can cause the band to slip, or it can cause reflux. It can also make band fills difficult to tolerate. The good news is that it can be fixed surgically.

Band intolerance. Some people just do not tolerate the band well; they may vomit excessively, even after a little fill, and they may feel very uncomfortable all the time. In these cases, the patient usually asks to have the band removed.

Band Versus Bypass

"I wasn't comfortable with someone moving my insides around, so I went with the band. I like the idea that it's reversible if I want it to be."

"I thought that as long as I was having the surgery, I might as well get the one that works fastest and helps you lose the most weight."

The question I'm most often asked in my practice is this one: "Between the band and the bypass, which surgery is best for me?"

Since I do both procedures, I think I have a pretty good perspective on the debate. Here are some of the pros and cons of both, as well as what I usually recommend to my patients.

The Band

Pros

It's flexible. We can increase the fill to speed your weight loss—or decrease it, to increase your nutrition. If you were to get pregnant or to get sick (cancer, for instance, requiring chemotherapy), we could just pull the fluid out of the band.

On the other hand, if you are eating too much, we can add fluid. I have even heard of a doctor removing the fluid from a patient who was going on a cruise. I personally wouldn't do this, but you get the idea—the band is adjustable.

It's reversible. If there's a problem or if you tolerate it poorly, we can simply take it out. No part of your stomach or intestine is cut or altered. Removal *is* a surgical procedure, but it's a pretty simple one.

There's no dumping syndrome. You can eat whatever you want, as long as you chew slowly to get it past the band.

Weight loss is slower, and it often takes place over a long period of time. Many of my band patients are still losing two and three years out—they've kept losing long after the bypass patients have leveled off, which may mean they lose less muscle.

(This can be frustrating in the beginning—especially if you go to a support group that includes bypass patients. They'll be talking about losing thirty pounds in a month while you're struggling to lose seven. The band does require persistence.)

There are very few serious complications with the band. Because we don't cut or divide the intestines, the risks for leaks, obstructions, ulcers, and vitamin deficiencies are very low.

Cons

There's less long-term data. The band is the new kid on the block. The version of the procedure that is most commonly used today was first performed in Europe in the 1990s; it has only been done in the United States since 2001.

We know that if you remove the band, you gain weight. What we do *not* know is how long the band will last (whether it will slip, start losing fluid, or erode into the stomach more frequently). Australian surgeons and researchers tell us that twelve years out, the band still works fine. As I mentioned earlier, though, at our international meetings, the Europeans tell us that many of their patients have the band removed at a later date for various reasons.

Weight loss with the band is slower, and you generally lose less weight than you would with the bypass. The Australians and the Belgians have published data over the years showing that the average weight loss with the band is 60 percent. The initial studies in the United States showed only a weight loss in the 30 to 40 percent range. This seemed much worse than the bypass, so a lot of weight-loss surgeons abandoned the band.

The problem turned out to be with the follow-up: The band needs to be carefully adjusted to just the right level of restriction, and the patient must be compliant—right off the bat—with the program of exercising and eating healthier foods. Since over the past five or so years, Americans have been doing more program-oriented weight loss—combining the band surgery with a comprehensive program of education and support and longer-term strategies, like the ones you'll find in this book—weight loss is now at about 50 to 55 percent on average in America's top centers.

I always point out to my patients that the band is a product, backed by a large company that makes a lot of money when you choose it. It stands to reason that they have a marketing team to get you to buy their product—and, of course, you know that advertising can be deceiving.

You may have seen ads for the band on television, on Web sites, and in magazines. They make it seem like it's a sure thing that you will lose 65 percent of your excess weight. But the fact is that the vast majority of American studies only show about 50 percent excess weight loss, and even this figure can be deceiving because it is just an average. There is a high standard of deviation with those studies, which means that you arrive at that 50 percent by combining people who only lose 20 percent with those who lose 80 percent.

In truth, I see a very broad range of response to the band. I have patients who do wonderfully and lose a lot of weight. These patients tend to be young, active, and not very obese to start with (a BMI from 35 to 45). But some don't respond as well; they keep eating junk food and they want the band tighter until it makes them vomit, but they still do not lose the weight. The tightest band in the world can't stop a milkshake.

Part of the problem may be that the band just doesn't work that well on hunger issues. One of the pros of the band is that we don't reroute the intestines, but it's also one of the cons. There's no hormonal effect, so my band patients tend to be hungrier than those who had the bypass. This isn't true for all of my band patients, of course, but it is true for some.

There's no dumping syndrome. The bad thing about dumping syndrome is that it makes you sick. The good thing about it is that it very effectively helps you to avoid high-sugar, high-fat foods—precisely the foods that will contribute to slow loss or even weight regain. If you have a sweet tooth or a taste for potato chips, it's easy to cheat on the band, and many people do, which certainly contributes to slower and less impressive weight-loss results.

You have a surgical device implanted in you. Some people simply don't like the idea of this. And, of course, the band can erode into the stomach, or it can slip, requiring another surgery to correct the problem.

The band takes more work on the patient's part. Because the band doesn't quell hunger as effectively as the bypass, band patients have to get serious about eating healthy foods and exercise as soon as they're out of surgery.

Getting the band fill exactly right—not too tight, not too loose—can be very difficult. One of my big concerns with the band is that making it tight enough for good weight loss often means making it too tight for good, healthy foods. The goal of all these surgeries is to get you eating a high-quality, healthful diet of whole foods. If the band is too tight, patients often find that this type of food—a piece of chicken breast and some snow peas, for instance—causes them discomfort, whereas chips and cookies, which can be crunched down to nothing, do not. The worst things for you, in other words, are the easiest to eat.

There are more frequent follow-ups. I see my band patients much more often than my bypass patients. We require monthly appointments during the six months immediately following the surgery, and fills whenever you feel hungrier, or you're not losing as much weight as you'd like. Sometimes the band takes a little noodling—a cc in, half a cc out—over several appointments to get the fill right.

The fills are done with a syringe. We use a topical anesthetic, and you don't have to watch, but I've had needlephobic patients choose bypass over band simply to eliminate this factor.

Problems with the band have to be resolved by someone familiar with the band. This is less of an issue every year, as more and more doctors become conversant with these surgeries and what needs to be done to maintain them. But if you regularly travel to the far corners of the earth, for work or for pleasure, the band might not be right for you. (Of course, if you watch the show, you know that my sister ran into trouble in Ohio—hardly a far corner!—and had problems finding someone who could deal with it. We ended up putting her on a plane and bringing her home.)

The Bypass

Pros

There's more long-term data. The bypass has been around for a while, so we have a good understanding of the risks, the benefits, and what to expect, even long-term.

The ghrelin factor. Because the part of the stomach that produces this appetite-promoting hormone is bypassed, this surgery really addresses hunger.

(The truth is, it may not just be ghrelin that kills hunger; we're learning that there are a host of hormones made by the intestines that are altered with the bypass. And this may be why the bypass is so immediately effective at eliminating diabetes; there's research that shows that the way food enters the intestine after bypass may increase certain hormones that create a feeling of fullness and help the body fight diabetes.)

You lose weight quickly, and you keep it off. We feel an operation is successful if you can lose 50 percent of your excess weight. The number of bypass patients that do not maintain this level of weight loss is said to be about 10 percent. So 90 percent of people have a successful result with bypass.

It is often said that bypass patients gain their weight back over time. It's true that there is a honeymoon period in the beginning where the weight just falls off, and that after a year or so, the bypass, like all weight-loss surgeries, becomes just a tool. However, that tool is very effective. While it is not uncommon to see some weight regain—from an 80 percent weight loss to 70 percent, say—patients generally keep the weight off.

Now, your neighbor may have had the surgery many years ago and gained back all of her weight. What's the story? One answer might lie in the fact that the bypass was done in many different ways in the past. We have learned that making a bigger pouch or a shorter Roux limb may negatively affect weight loss. And yet Dr. Walter Pories, one of the fathers of weight-loss surgery, who followed his bypass patients for fifteen years, was using a shorter Roux limb in the 80s and a bigger pouch, but even many years out, his bypass patients had still kept off 50 percent of their excess weight.

We're seeing even better numbers with our newer techniques. The way we perform the bypass now, it is very difficult *not* to lose weight and keep it off.

Cons

There is a risk of malnutrition and vitamin deficiency. After the bypass, you have to agree to take supplements—iron, B_{12}, calcium, and a multivitamin—for the rest of your life or run the risk of serious deficiencies. You also have to focus on getting between 60 and 80 grams of protein a day or risk malnutrition. You also have to return to your surgeon's office to be checked for deficiencies at least once a year.

Complications. Bypass is a more serious surgery than the band, and the attendant problems tend to be more involved, even if they're rarer. I feel that weight-loss surgeons perform the bypass in a way that is very safe for the majority of people, but, as discussed earlier, serious complications can occur, including leaks, bowel obstructions, ulcers, and vitamin deficiency.

Dumping syndrome (see page 134). Dumping syndrome is the bypassed stomach's reaction to high-sugar (and sometimes high-fat) foods. While it does effectively keep you away from these foods, which is certainly a boon to your weight loss, it's unpleasant and not always avoidable.

It's irreversible. The bypass can be reversed, but it's a difficult procedure, and one with many more complications than the original surgery. Unless there's a serious medical reason to do it, it should be avoided; I advise my patients to regard this surgery as permanent.

That's the overview. And if it seems like I lean toward the bypass, you're not wrong.

Here's what I often tell my patients who are on the fence: My bypass patients tend to be *happier* with their surgeries and with their results.

They're less hungry, and the weight comes off easier. They tend to have fewer of the minor difficulties that make life unpleasant on a daily basis—the sensation of something getting stuck, the gurgling, the sudden vomiting—than people with the band. A bypass patient a year out can almost forget they had anything done, but I've seen a lot of people struggle with tolerating the band.

My bypass patients also do seem to be more successful in the long run. As I say in my seminars, I find that I can very reliably predict the weight loss of bypass patients—they will lose about 75 percent of their excess weight, gain a bit back, and then stabilize.

That prediction is more difficult with band patients. As I've said, the 50 percent average weight loss really is an average. Some of my patients lose a ton of weight (in the 70 percent range), keep it off, and go dancing. Others struggle with old eating habits and exercise and only lose 20 percent. To go through a surgical procedure and the fills and everything else just to lose 20 percent of excess weight—20 pounds for someone who is a 100 pounds overweight—is a very disappointing outcome. We do work closely with people to help them get their diet, exercise, and mind-set on track so that they see the weight loss they want to see, but it's a struggle for them.

I know that some of my very successful band patients will want to kill me when they read this. They love their band and would have the surgery all over again in a second. If you watch *Big Medicine*, you know that my sister has problems tolerating her band at times; in fact, it can make her very ill indeed. But she is thrilled with her weight loss, and she has made me promise that I would never ever take it out. She gets very mad if she hears me say a bad word about it.

Deciding which surgery is right for you is something that deserves careful consideration—and careful discussion with your doctor. As you'll see from just a quick review of Web sites such as ObesityHelp.com, people are passionate about their choice! The more you read and research—and the better you know yourself—the better equipped you'll be to determine the procedure best suited to you. (We'll talk more about whether or not weight loss surgery in general is the right path for you in the next chapter.)

BAND VERSUS BYPASS
A Summary

Choose the band if:

You are young and not too overweight, without many co-morbidities.
You have osteoporosis or an iron deficiency or anemia.
You are prone to ulcers or have had tumors in your stomach.
You have serious health issues, such as severe heart disease, cancer that may recur, or chronic debilitating illnesses.

Choose the bypass if:

You have diabetes. (There was a recent *Journal of American Medicine* article that showed pretty impressive diabetes control with the band, but it's still not nearly as good as the bypass for resolving diabetes.)
You're older.
You are very overweight, with a BMI in the 50s or above.
You tend to be a binge eater or sweets eater.

Note that these are just guidelines; my colleagues and I honor any decision a patient makes and do our best to help make that procedure work for him or her. No matter which one you go with, please remember:

Both surgeries are just tools.

Neither will be successful if you're not dedicated to exercising regularly and eating small portions of high-quality, healthy foods. Band patients have to learn to use their tool immediately; bypass patients enjoy a honeymoon period for the first year to eighteen months, but they, too, have to learn to exercise and eat correctly.

The band and the bypass are the most common options. But there are other weight-loss surgeries as well, including:

Biliopancreatic Diversion, or Duodenal Switch (BPD/DS)

This procedure is similar to the gastric bypass. It's generally performed only in the super-obese, although there are surgeons out there who do this surgery regularly.

I personally do not perform this surgery, mainly because the risks are substantial, and because I think that a bypass done with a good aftercare program can be just as successful. But the DS is a very effective surgery, particularly if you are very overweight (with a BMI above 60).

The procedure. First, instead of creating a small roundish stomach pouch, the surgeon creates a sleeve-shaped stomach by removing about 75 percent of the stomach (this part of the procedure is called a sleeve gastrectomy).

Next—instead of cutting the intestine high up, at the jejunum—the intestine is divided low down, about 100 cm from the colon. We then bring the intestine up and join it to the reduced (but not tiny) stomach. As a result, only a 100 cm of small intestine receives food combined with digestive juices, which means that only 100 cm of small bowel is able to absorb calories.

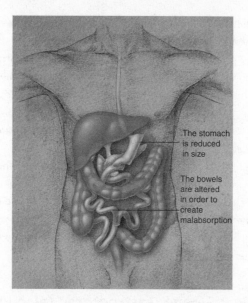

The stomach is reduced in size

The bowels are altered in order to create malabsorption

How it works. This surgery is very similar to that first weight-loss surgery I described earlier, the JI bypass, in that it is primarily malabsorptive. There is some restriction from the reduced-size stomach, but this surgery works primarily by restricting the amount of food/calories that can be *absorbed*. (The gastric bypass, as it is currently done, works mainly by restricting *meal size*.) Also, as with the bypass, there are many hormonal changes, too, that help to control hunger.

The results are impressive: Weight loss with the DS generally is higher than with the bypass in almost all studies.

The risks. If the DS is the best surgery for weight loss, you're probably wondering why I don't perform this procedure. The main reason is that the risks are much higher.

The surgery itself is much more dangerous than the bypass because there's more bowel bypassed, and the connections are more difficult to make. As a result, it comes with many of the same risks—leaks, bowel obstruction, bleeding, and all the rest, but there is a higher rate of occurrence in each category. It takes longer to perform the surgery, so the patient is under anesthesia for quite some time. And the mortality rate is worse. A patient's risk of dying with a bypass is generally less than 0.5 percent, while the DS has a 0.8 to 1.5 percent risk of death.

But the real problem for me with the DS is the malabsorption. Frequent diarrhea is common, and patients may also have problems absorbing enough protein and vitamins, which can lead to anemia due to problems with iron absorption, osteoporosis due to calcium and vitamin D malabsorption, night blindness due to vitamin A malabsorption, and several other vitamin and mineral deficiencies.

The DS definitely has its place for the severely obese individual, but it should only be done by experienced surgeons who have a comprehensive program, and there aren't many around. In fact, at the time of this writing, in Houston there are no programs offering the DS. So if you are severely obese and considering a DS, be sure that you search for someone with extensive experience in this procedure.

Vertical Sleeve Gastrectomy (also known as the Sleeve Gastrectomy or Vertical Gastrectomy)

If you attend one of my seminars, you'll hear me ask who in the audience will be paying for the procedure themselves because they don't have insurance coverage.

Then you'll hear me tell everyone else to cover their ears.

Here's why: The sleeve gastrectomy is quickly becoming my favorite surgery to recommend. The problem? It's not covered by insurance. It's too new, and with too little long-term data to support its use. I recently attended an international conference on the sleeve gastrectomy where we reviewed the research data from around the world. The consensus was that this surgery works. Hopefully the insurance companies will listen. But in the meantime, I feel like I'm just torturing people by tempting them with a procedure they can't get unless they pay for it.

The history of this operation is actually pretty interesting. Bypass surgery on people with a BMI over 60 is very dangerous, so surgeons wondered if there was another, safer operation that could be done *first*—before a bypass. The procedure that they came up with was the sleeve gastrectomy. The idea was that once the patient had lost some weight from the sleeve gastrectomy, he or she could come back for a bypass. But surgeons all over the world began reporting that their sleeve gastrectomy patients were doing very well—as well, if not better, than their bypass patients. A lot of them never went back to do the second stage—the bypass—at all.

What's not to love? It's a lower-risk surgery than the bypass, with similar results. Granted, it's still pretty uncommon; not very many surgeons perform it, and even fewer people can pay for it. But I, personally, think it's the wave of the future.

The procedure. During the sleeve gastrectomy, the stomach is divided vertically, creating a long, skinny pouch about the size and shape of a banana. We do this by placing a tube down your mouth while you are under anesthesia. This tube is about as wide as your thumb and passes all the way through your stomach. We then put our surgical stapler against the tube and staple up the stomach around it; finally, we remove the excess stomach through one of the small laparoscopic holes.

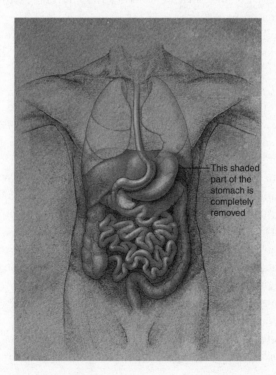

This shaded part of the stomach is completely removed

How it works. Like the bypass, the section of the stomach that is removed is the part responsible for secreting ghrelin, the hormone that drives hunger. The remaining stomach is considerably smaller, of course, just as it is with the pouch in the bypass, and it also happens to be the section of the stomach that stretches the least. With the bypass, the remaining stomach holds about 20 cc, which is about 4 ounces of food. With the sleeve, the remaining stomach is larger—about 150 cc—but you still get full with about 4 ounces of food. This may be due to the hormones, but it is also because food in the small tube creates a pressure that makes you feel full.

Why I like it. First of all, it's a simpler surgery; since we don't mess with the intestine, there are considerably fewer complications. Bowel obstruction does not happen, there is no dumping, and we haven't seen much in the way of nutritional deficiency. (I do have my patients take a multivitamin, because they're eating much less, making it harder to obtain a balanced diet; I also have them supplement with B_{12}, because part of the stomach that is removed may be used to absorb it.) There's also a reduced risk of ulcer afterward.

Best of all, the early data (and my own observations of the patients on which I've done the surgery) are reporting weight loss results that are close to what we see with the bypass.

Risks

We are still stapling the stomach; with that comes a risk of bleeding, leaks, and infection. These risks generally are lower than with the bypass, but when they do occur, they are handled much the same way.

Some patients do have some nausea in the beginning. As with the bypass, this usually passes with time. Also, the tube can stricture, like the bypass, and need to be dilated.

Some patients have described reflux with the sleeve, but this can usually be handled with good eating techniques and the occasional antacid.

My biggest worry with the sleeve is long-term weight regain. We just do not have enough evidence yet proving that the "sleeve" we create will not expand. In fact, some surgeons have already described this happening in their patients. They have treated this by going back in and cutting the stomach back down to size or by converting the surgery to a bypass.

Generally speaking, weight loss looks to be about 50 to 55 percent of excess weight at five years with the sleeve gastrectomy, but we need more data to prove it.

What Else Is Out There?

The band and the bypass have become so safe and effective that they have really set the bar. There are older surgeries for weight loss and additional ideas for new surgeries, but none have yet been able to rival these two procedures—although I feel that the sleeve gastrectomy will be another serious player once the insurance companies get on board. You may find the following procedures being discussed in the course of your research, though, so I'll give you a brief rundown:

Vertical Banded Gastroplasty

As I've already mentioned, years ago, doctors tried all kinds of stomach stapling procedures. The Vertical Banded Gastroplasty, or VBG, was the predominant surgery of the 80s and 90s. It is still done today by some surgeons, but given the fact that it results in less weight loss than the bypass and more complications than the band, it has been practically abandoned as a viable procedure.

Gastric Pacing

Within the weight-loss surgery community, for a while there was a theory that if you surgically connected pacing wires to a nerve in the stomach connected to the part of the brain that controls satiety and then sent electrical signals to that nerve, the patient would not get hungry. The trials were very disappointing. Some patients did well, but most did not lose weight. This is not offered anymore.

The Balloon (also called the BIB)

This procedure has been studied extensively recently. It involves passing a balloon into the stomach through the mouth using a scope. The balloon is then blown up, making the patient feel full all the time, like you just ate a huge hamburger—or swallowed a balloon.

This can be pretty uncomfortable, and vomiting is frequent. In general, it's just not well tolerated, and it doesn't result in great weight loss.

The Mini Gastric Bypass

Don't be fooled by the name; it's an advertising gimmick—there's nothing mini about it. I won't dignify it with further detail; suffice to say, there is no benefit to this procedure, and indeed, there may be more risk. My advice is to ignore the catchy name and stick with the tried and true.

Endoscopic (or Incisionless) Weight-Loss Procedures

This is also called NOTES (Natural Orifice Transluminal Endoscopic Surgery). It's a complex procedure that involves making the stomach smaller using a scope from the mouth into the stomach without actually making any incisions. It is highly experimental at this time and not yet ready for prime time now, and likely not in the near future.

When Weight-Loss Surgery Doesn't Work

Revision Surgery

As you now know, weight-loss surgery has evolved over the years, and many surgeries have come and gone. It stands to reason, then, that there are many people out there stuck with surgeries that aren't very effective or that cause complications down the line. So my father and I are often faced with the need to "revise" a prior weight-loss surgery.

Please note: Effective diet and exercise are essential to success, no matter what kind of surgery you've had. No doctor will revise a perfectly good surgery that's not working simply because you're not following the game plan.

**In order to have a revision,
there should be something functionally wrong
with the original surgery.**

A revision will convert an ineffective surgery into one that works. But risks are always increased with a revision. The scar tissue from old surgeries can make the tissues very thick, and the result is invariably a longer and more dangerous surgery.

Revising the bypass. The bypass has been done many different ways over the years: Some surgeons made too big a pouch, while others left a part of the stomach that is very stretchy and expandable. (We've discovered that both of these factors can result in inadequate weight loss.)

If patients are not losing enough weight after a bypass, I generally will first ask them to keep a very accurate food diary. I like patients to use Fit-Day.com, a free online food journal that allows us to determine a patient's exact calorie intake (it also accounts for exercise expenditure). Also, our dietician will have them breathe into a special machine that allows us to calculate their basal metabolic expenditure, which is the amount of calories their bodies burn in a day. Then we can see exactly how many surplus calories they are eating, and the dietician can design a meal plan that puts the patient back into calorie deficit (assuming he or she isn't already).

I also have the patient meet with our psychotherapist. While the bypass is good at controlling physiologic hunger, it does not take care of hunger that happens because you are bored, depressed, or stressed. Our fantastic therapist, Mary Jo Rapini, who you may have seen on *Big Medicine*, helps people understand why they are sabotaging their success, and she gives them behavioral techniques to change their habits. (We'll talk more about this later.)

If none of this works, I will take a closer look at the bypass itself, using three different tests. The first is a procedure called an upper GI, which requires you to drink a dye while getting X-rays so I can see your pouch. Next, I'll do an endoscopy so I can actually see the size of the pouch and the size of the opening of the stomach to the intestine. The final test is a little more low-tech; we have you eat cottage cheese until you're full, and then see how much you ate. If you have had a bypass and you can eat 8 to 10 ounces of cottage cheese and the scope and upper GI study show a large pouch, a revision may be beneficial to make the pouch smaller.

Some surgeons advocate placing a band around the existing pouch. There is anecdotal evidence that this can be successful, but not enough scientific evidence to prove its safety and efficacy. I still view this as experimental and would prefer to cut the pouch down in size rather than place the band.

There are new procedures out there now that allow us to make the pouch smaller using a device that is passed through the mouth into the pouch. One version is called StomaphyX, which basically creates pleats on the inside of the pouch, narrowing it and the outlet. This is a very new and very experimental procedure. I like the fact that there is no cutting involved, and it does seem to be very safe, but there is very little data regarding its efficacy.

Some people believe that the size of the outlet of the pouch determines weight loss; I don't. I have patients with huge openings who have lost lots of weight—and others with tiny openings who have not lost as much. There are procedures to make the outlet smaller, but I do not perform them because I don't believe they work.

Finally, there is the occasional patient with a small pouch and good compliance with the program but an amazingly low metabolic rate. The best thing these patients can do is to speed up their metabolism by exercising. Some surgeons will offer to lengthen the Roux, which has the effect of converting the bypass, a mainly restrictive procedure, to a surgery that is similar to the DS, a mainly malabsorptive surgery. While this is effective for weight loss, it carries all the risks listed in the DS section above.

Revision of the band. Some people can't tolerate the band; others develop a hiatal hernia that makes filling the band very difficult, and sometimes the band slips.

If the problem is weight loss, a thorough nutritional and psychological evaluation needs to be done. We must also make sure that the band is adequately filled and is not leaking. It is easy to check for a leak: We just measure the amount of fluid we put in and make sure we can withdraw the same amount. If there's no leak, we will do an upper GI so I can be sure that the band is adequately tight.

The band is pretty easy to remove; many patients opt to have their band converted to a bypass. Like any other revision, it is more dangerous than if we were doing the bypass as a primary procedure because of the scar tissue where the band was attached to the stomach; that tissue is thicker, and it can be difficult to staple.

If the band has slipped or there is a hiatal hernia, we can go back in and fix the band position and the hiatal hernia without the need to switch to a bypass. In some patients with the older band, I will switch them to the newer bands, called AP Allergan bands, which I think are better tolerated.

Revision of the duodenal switch. It is very uncommon to have to do a revision on a DS for inadequate weight loss. It's more likely that a revision would be required because the patient is losing too much weight or experiencing diarrhea or vitamin deficiency.

The DS revision is done by cutting the intestines and rearranging them so that food gets to mix with the digestive juices earlier and can travel through a longer piece of intestine so that more of it is absorbed.

Revision of the sleeve gastrectomy. With this procedure, the sleeved stomach can grow over time, which can result in weight gain. This can be documented by an X-ray study, and it can be revised by re-sleeving the stomach. We put the tube back down into the stomach and cut along that tube to remove the excess stomach. It is also fairly simple to switch the sleeve into a bypass by cutting the sleeve where we would have made a pouch for the bypass, and bringing up a piece of intestine to connect.

We may also revise a sleeve to a bypass if the patient is suffering from reflux; the bypass is a great treatment for reflux.

Revision of a vertical banded gastroplasty. The VBG was a very popular surgery in the 80s and 90s, so this is a very common revision. One-third to half of patients fail with the VBG or suffer from severe reflux or vomiting caused by the band at the end of the chamber. We can revise to a bypass by cutting across and up the chamber, creating a pouch, and then bringing up a piece of intestine. These revisions can be very difficult and dangerous to perform, and there is an increased risk of leak.

I do not see as much weight loss with revision patients. This may be because the prior procedure has stretched out the top part of the stomach or because we are dealing with people who have failed one weight-loss surgery and have poor eating and exercise habits. Despite this, I've revised many people, and most are very happy with their results.

CHAPTER FIVE

Is Weight-Loss Surgery Right for Me?

"You only get one shot at life, and I finally realized that life in a size 32 was not the one I wanted for myself."

"Losing the weight just wasn't something I could do for myself. I'd tried everything; if I could have, I would have. I needed help, and I got it."

Being a good candidate for weight-loss surgery entails more than being able to satisfy medical criteria. These surgeries are not a quick fix, and they will require a real commitment to change. In this chapter, I'll try to help you answer seven very important questions, including this big one: Is weight loss surgery right for *you*?

1) Are you morbidly obese?

Medical criteria might not be all of it, but it's certainly a good place to start. The National Institutes of Health decided that bariatric surgery was appropriate for people who were 100 pounds or more above an ideal body weight or who had a BMI of 35 or more.

The insurance companies have modified this, and they require that you have a BMI of above 40 or a serious co-morbidity and a BMI between 35 and 40.

There is a movement afoot to drop the BMI cutoff to 30. There are surgeons who will do bands on patients with a BMI of 30 to 35, and they have published very good results. The conference held in Rome to discuss how weight-loss can cure diabetes produced a consensus hinting that weight-loss surgery, including bypass, is probably appropriate for these patients if they have diabetes.

Most surgeons stick to a cutoff of 35, and insurance companies absolutely will not pay if your BMI is less than 35.

WHAT ABOUT KIDS?

Are children good candidates for weight-loss surgery?

It's a good question; certainly childhood obesity is a pressing issue, as it is growing at astronomical rates. Type 2 diabetes, which is strongly correlated to obesity, used to be known as adult-onset diabetes until the growing number of children with this disease forced a nomenclature change. The patient liaison at my practice, Jamie Carr, interviewed Dr. Richard Carmona, the former surgeon general of the United States, for a publication called *WLS Lifestyles* a few years ago. In it, Dr. Carmona said something that sent a chill down my spine: Rising obesity rates among children may mean that we are the first generation in history whose children have a shorter life expectancy than our own.

Certainly we must pay attention to the eating behaviors we model for our children; in fact, one of the collateral benefits I notice in families where one (or both) parents have had WLS is that *everyone* gets healthier. Getting the junk out of the house doesn't just help patients stay compliant; it's the best thing for their kids.

But as we know, obesity is, at least in part, a genetic disorder. In many cases, these children are already seriously obese by a very young age—and exhibiting co-morbidities usually associated with much older people while they're still in their teens. So what about using WLS as a way to treat obese kids and teens? Some surgeons say that adolescents should not have surgery because they may outgrow their obesity. Unfortunately, that's not what we see: Instead, more than 75 percent of obese children become obese adults.

I think that weight-loss surgery may provide us with a partial solution to the epidemic rise in childhood obesity, but with a few caveats. First, our priority has to be making sure that children get adequate nutrition so that they continue to grow properly. Doctors consider growth to be finished when the growth plates in the bones are fully fused, which usually takes place around puberty or a little later. (A pediatrician can do an X-ray to determine if the growth plates have fused.) I would not recommend these surgeries for anyone whose plates haven't yet fused.

The other big concern for me when contemplating these surgeries for kids is the issue of compliance. With either surgery, you must learn to eat healthfully and to exercise daily. After the bypass in particular, it is imperative that you get adequate protein and that you take supplements religiously. It is also essential to return to the doctor often for follow-up blood tests in order to make sure you're not suffering from a deficiency. Obviously, this takes a lot of discipline—discipline that, frankly, a lot of young people don't yet have. For these reasons, the band is often considered a better procedure for young people.

It is imperative for me to ensure that an adolescent patient not only has a good understanding of the postsurgical requirements but also a strongly supportive family dynamic so that those requirements would be met. I certainly require preoperative participation in our nutrition classes and sessions with our psychotherapist.

That said, adolescents are at a crucial time for the development of their social skills, and being obese during those years can seriously affect their future. Adolescents heal fast and have fewer complications than adults do— and they lose a lot of weight. I think it is better to prevent diseases from occurring prematurely than to wait until a young person is already suffering.

2) Can you lose weight another way and keep it off?

Weight-loss surgery is a treatment of last resort, which is to say that it's for people who have tried unsuccessfully to lose weight through conventional methods. If you haven't tried a medically supervised diet and exercise program, you should explore those options before taking this step.

If you have tried diets and exercise, it's worth examining what happened and why these approaches failed you in the past. When patients see a dietician for the first time, they are usually asked about their diet history in a questionnaire that looks something like this:

- When did you become obese (in childhood, when you hit puberty, as an adult)?

- If you have not always been obese, was there an event that led to your weight gain (a pregnancy, a divorce, an injury or medical condition, job loss, the death of a parent, and so on)?

- When was the first time you went (or were put) on a diet?

- Have you tried to lose weight using diet and exercise? Use this space to list your attempts. Include diets you've tried as well as weight-loss attempts that were medically supervised. Did you lose weight? How long were you able to maintain that loss?

- Have you used medication in order to help you lose weight? Which ones?

If you decide to go through with the surgery, it's crucial that you don't bring feelings of "diet failure" into it with you. This time you will have the tools you need to succeed.

In order to best take advantage of these tools, however, in the months leading up to the procedure, you'll want to investigate the stumbling blocks you faced with conventional dieting and exercise; issues like emotional eating or poor habits can interfere with your best progress after surgery if they're not addressed. This is why we require all prospective patients to meet with our dieticians and psychologists preoperatively.

And if you do have unresolved issues stemming from a traumatic event, I recommend getting counseling in order to deal with that as well.

We'll talk more about preparing for the surgery in Chapter 8.

DO AFRICAN AMERICANS LOSE LESS WEIGHT?

Yes—slightly. According to a study published in *Obesity Surgery*, African American people *do* lose less weight after weight-loss surgery than their Caucasian counterparts. The reasons for this were not fully explored; the authors of the paper recommend further research into the possible genetic and social reasons for the discrepancy.

The study found that African American participants lost 66 percent of their excess weight, as compared to the 74 percent lost by the Caucasian participants. As you know, losing 66 percent of your excess weight is still a pretty great result, and one that's going to make an enormous difference in a person's general health. My conclusion is that, even with the discrepancy, weight-loss surgery is a good option for everyone.

3) Are you highly motivated to lose weight?

I often suggest that my patients make a list of the factors that are motivating them. This is helpful, not only in gearing up for surgery, but later, when they hit a rough patch and need a little motivation.

Take a piece of paper and write down your reasons for contemplating this surgery. Reasons might include wanting to look better, wanting to wear different kinds of clothes, or wanting relief from physical conditions caused by obesity. You might want to have more freedom to travel, or to have more energy for your relationship, your job, or your kids. This is for your eyes only: Be honest about what you're looking forward to shedding along with those pounds—and to gaining when you're on the losing side.

4) Will you be able to comply with the postsurgical requirements?

"Oh, you lost all that weight, but you didn't really have to do anything." That's something weight-loss patients often hear, and it makes the steam come out of their ears when they do. Perhaps the most common—and annoying—misconception about weight-loss surgery is that it somehow represents "the easy way out."

In fact, a great deal will be required of you. Yes, the weight will come off, and no, you won't be hungry the way you were on diets in the past. But in order for you to see the best results, and to see them over the long term, you will have to commit to a diet, exercise, and supplementation program, as well as medical follow-ups, *for the rest of your life*. It is a tremendous amount of work, which is why it's not a decision to be taken lightly.

Before I operate on a patient, I need to know that they really, really understand what they're in for. That's why you have to answer the following question honestly:

**Can you commit to making healthy dietary,
exercise, and medical choices over the rest of your
lifetime?**

The simple truth is that weight-loss surgery is not a replacement for behavior modification. Without behavior modification, your weight-loss surgery will not work as well.

5) Do you have the support of your family?

"It was a big adjustment for all of us—bigger than I'd thought it would be. I couldn't have done it without them; I'm glad they were on board."

"If I could have one thing different, it would be more support from my husband and kids. It's been a struggle to get time to exercise and to keep unhealthy food out of the house."

The people who have the most support are the ones who are most likely to be successful. In general, I find that family members tend to be very supportive because they have an up-close and personal understanding of the physical and social challenges faced by people suffering from obesity, and they're willing to do whatever it takes to help their loved ones to feel better. In many cases, they're the ones who did the primary research and made the suggestion of weight-loss surgery in the first place.

The support of your family is essential. Don't forget: Although you're the one going through all the changes, the effects of your surgery will ripple outward and affect everyone in your life. You'll need physical help in the days immediately after the surgery and someone to pick up the slack domestically, whether that means taking care of your kids, the pets, or the house.

But that's really only the tip of the iceberg. The types of foods you'll be eating and the portions in which you'll be eating them will change drastically after the surgery, and your family members will have to be educated in your new ways. You wouldn't believe how many calls I get from family members: "Billy's not eating enough!" Most people think it is normal and healthy to eat a 12-ounce steak, french fries, an ear of corn, and dessert, so if they haven't been with you through all the preoperative training, they certainly will think that a 4-ounce meal is not enough. Grocery shopping will be different; going out for dinner will be different. *You'll* be different. And that can be disorienting for family members.

What if you meet resistance? When family members aren't immediately supportive of your decision to look into surgery, I generally find that education is the solution. Media reports about these surgeries can be very frightening; if someone I loved wanted one of these surgeries, and all I knew was what I'd learned from the eleven o'clock news, I'd be terrified, too!

They may also be afraid of what the change in you will bring. If your family traditionally bonds over home cooking, what's going to happen when you have to say no to lasagna? Your spouse may be worried about what happens after you lose the weight. What will you do together if you're not eating? Will you still find him or her attractive? Will others find *you* attractive in a way that threatens them? Your kids may have concerns about you going into the hospital, and they may be worried that you'll end up different from the mom or dad they've always known—a very frightening prospect for a child, as you might imagine.

So you may have to make the case to your family, just as you would for anyone else. Talk to them about how your obesity affects your life—socially, emotionally, and medically. Show them information on the potential risks. Sometimes it can help to talk to someone together, whether that's a counselor or a clergyperson or just a trusted friend. Often spouses accompany patients to their early appointments with me. I welcome the opportunity to answer their questions—sometimes they have more of them than the person who's having the surgery! One of the most helpful things you can do is to take your spouse with you to support group meetings. That way, he or she can see just what postoperative patients face and the kinds of changes they go through.

Most of all, you'll have to make clear to your family what the benefits will be—for all of you. You'll have more energy, more self-confidence, and you'll live longer!

GOING AHEAD WITHOUT THEIR GO-AHEAD

I've only operated on a handful of people who were having the operation against the wishes of their family members. It's hardly an ideal situation, but, ultimately, this is your health, and your decision. If your surgeon and you agree that you're a good candidate, and you haven't had success in losing weight another way, you may decide to proceed, even without the blessing of your family.

No matter what, though, it's not a good idea to go it alone.

If you are having this surgery without the support of your immediate family, you'll need to find support somewhere else.

Ask your friends if they're willing to step in to help in the days immediately after surgery. The weight-loss surgery community is another amazing resource, filled with people who are more than happy to help out someone who's just starting out; ask your surgeon if a previous patient might be willing to be your "angel," accompanying you to your appointments and helping you get ready for surgery, or look in the online weight-loss surgery groups for someone in your area who'd be willing to help. And make sure you have a really good support system set up for afterward, including a bariatric support group and possibly some individual counseling. Every weight-loss surgery patient needs these tools, but without the support of your family, you may need to lean even more heavily on them.

And don't lose hope. Once your family members see how much healthier and happier you are, they may very well come around.

6) Does your doctor consider you to be a good candidate?

The NIH and insurance guidelines aren't the only medical guidelines you'll have to satisfy; many surgical practices have their own measures of eligibility and won't operate on those who don't meet them.

For instance, a practice might require that patients:

- Be ambulatory. People confined to bed or wheelchairs have a much higher risk of blood clots. I do not personally require that people are walking, but surgery is both riskier and less successful if the patient cannot be active afterward.

- Be below a BMI of 50. As BMI increases, so do the risks. We do not have a size cutoff, and we will do the surgeries on larger patients, but we'll also work with patients who have a BMI over 50 to help them lose weight in the months leading up to the surgery. Typically we require all our patients with a BMI greater than 50 to lose 10 percent of their weight prior to surgery in order to make it safer.

- Be under a certain age. Studies have shown that the risk-benefit ratio for these surgeries changes pretty dramatically in older pa-tients, which is to say that they get more dangerous—and less efficacious—after the age of sixty-five. For that reason, many sur-geons don't operate on older people. This is a hotly debated topic. Some people say the band is better than the bypass for older people because it is less risky—but it is also less effective. Personally, I think that if you are fairly fit, the bypass is an option up to about seventy years old.

Here are some other reasons why your doctor may conclude that you're not an ideal candidate:

- There are medical conditions that increase risks, such as clotting disorders, lupus, and connective tissue disorders. In patients with cancer or chronic diseases, I will offer a band but usually not a by-pass, and then only if those diseases are controlled.

- I often get patients coming to me for weight loss so they can qualify for kidney transplant. Usually I will only do a band in these cases, because the meds patients must take after the transplant can cause an ulcer.

- Patients with Crohn's disease or ulcerative colitis cannot have weight-loss surgery. Occasionally I will consider a band for a controlled ulcerative colitis patient, but definitely not a patient with Crohn's, because Crohn's can affect the stomach.

- Patients with arthritis stand to benefit from weight-loss surgery, but if considering a bypass, they must know that most arthritis pain medications (NSAIDs) can cause an ulcer in the pouch and should not be taken after surgery.

- I require a cardiac clearance in all patients over fifty, or in any patient who is diabetic, has had chest pain, or has both high blood pressure and high cholesterol. It's easy to get into a catch-22 with cardiac issues: A patient with very bad congestive heart failure definitely would be better after losing weight, but the condition may make the surgery too risky. These are things you have to discuss with your surgeon.

- Prior surgeries can interfere with patient selection. If you have had many hernia surgeries, it may become difficult to get into your abdomen. The same thing is true about the scar tissue that comes about after intestinal surgery. Often a band is a better option in these situations because with a band we don't need to touch the intestines. I spoke about revisions of prior weight-loss suvrgeries being difficult, but surgery in patients who have undergone stomach wraps for reflux, also called hiatal hernia repairs, or Nissen Fundoplication (stomach wrap), are even more difficult, especially for the band and the bypass; a DS is a possibility if you can find someone who performs them.

As disappointed as you may be when a surgeon tells you you're not a good candidate, you shouldn't argue; you don't want a doctor to do something outside his or her comfort level. If you get a no from a surgeon, ask if there's a procedure that would be safe for you. If not, ask if the surgeon knows a doctor who might be willing to operate on you; some practices specialize in difficult cases.

7) Are your expectations realistic?

"I didn't realize how different life would be in this new body. Mostly good, but not all good."

"If I had to tell candidates one thing, it would be: Losing weight isn't going to solve all your problems!"

I've seen lots of "befores" and "afters." In my experience, knowing the cold, hard facts about what you can realistically expect after surgery—even if those facts aren't exactly what you want to hear—is a better route than rose-colored glasses.

I always feel like a buzz-kill introducing these concepts, especially given how happy most of my patients find themselves after surgery. (Remember, 95 percent of weight-loss surgery patients report a significant improvement in their quality of life.) But I think it's important to talk about these things while patients are still contemplating the procedure so that they make an informed choice.

It won't be easy. It's very tempting to think of the surgery as a magical cure. But, in fact, success requires a tremendous amount of effort, education, and determination on the part of the patient. The road ahead won't be easy. In fact, some days won't be fun at all.

Results won't be immediate. You'll wake up in the recovery room and you'll feel completely different, but you'll look exactly the same, and you will for a while. It probably will take about a year and half for you to end up at your "final" weight with a bypass, and longer with the band.

Your relationships may change. Your best friend may have a hard time with the fact that she's not "the thin one" anymore. Your spouse may feel less secure in the relationship. Other people may feel judged by your new portion sizes or by the way you wear your new clothes. Some of these relationships will recontour themselves to accommodate "the new you"—but, unfortunately, others might not survive.

Surgery won't change your relationship to food; *you* have to change your relationship to food. Surgery will give you a number of tools—a smaller stomach and reduced hunger—that can help you work through your food feelings more effectively than you've ever been able to before. But the procedure won't fix your relationship to food.

And an unresolved unhealthy relationship with food is as sure a road to trouble after surgery as it is before. Some people fall into a terrible, potentially dangerous depression when their primary emotional crutch—food—is "taken away" by the surgery. Others transfer their addiction to food to something else—shopping, sex, drugs, or alcohol. Others take their eating disorder in the opposite direction, eating much too little instead of much too much.

With dedication and help, you can put these feelings in their proper place and learn to use food as fuel. But you will need to dedicate yourself to that process, and perhaps be open to getting some help.

There will be challenges along the way. You'll hit plateaus, or times when the weight won't come off, even though you're doing everything right. You may gain a little bit of weight after you've reached your goal weight and before you stabilize—most of my patients do. There will be days when you hear that chocolate milkshake calling out to you. Those are all challenges that you'll have to push through. Support will be important; so will a continued commitment to your goals.

Even after all is said and done, you may not look like a supermodel. Everywhere we look, we see images of "perfect bodies"—men with washboard stomachs and 0 percent body fat; bikini-clad women without an ounce of cellulite or self-consciousness.

I'm hardly the first person to note that this puts a tremendous amount of pressure on "ordinary" people, or to complain that the emphasis in too many cases is more on looking good than feeling healthy. But I do hear my patients struggling with these issues after surgery, and I wonder if the perfect-body culture doesn't have an even more acute impact on the formerly obese than it does on everyone else. When people are obese, they feel completely shut out from a society that puts toned arms and thinner thighs above all else. But even after massive, life-extending weight loss, they still may find themselves disappointed by their quest for that "perfect" body.

You're going to look much better—no, you're going to look terrific. And you're going to feel amazing, compared to what you're used to feeling like now. But it's important to realize that, even at the end of your journey, you still may not be catwalk-ready. You still may be carrying some excess weight—remember, the average is 65 to 75 percent, not 100 percent—and you also may be left with excess skin.

I think you can learn to love that new, healthier body. Do you?

|||||||||||

Ultimately, the message I give to my patients who are deciding whether or not to pursue surgery is this:

Weight-loss surgery won't change your life.
But if you want to change your life,
weight-loss surgery can help.

Take the time to think carefully about it. Talk to your family and to your friends. Go to a support group. Many welcome preop patients; after all, everyone in that room was once in your shoes. And don't overlook the Internet as a resource—although you definitely should take what you find there with a grain of salt.

If, after this soul-searching, you feel that you are indeed a good candidate for this surgery, congratulations. It's time to find a doctor.

CHAPTER SIX

‖‖‖‖‖‖‖‖‖‖‖‖‖‖‖‖‖‖‖‖‖‖‖‖‖‖‖‖‖‖‖‖‖‖‖‖

Finding a Doctor

Finding the right surgeon—and surgical practice—is the next step you'll take toward surgery, and it's an important one.

Above all, you want to have paramount confidence in your surgeon's technique. But you also want to feel comfortable with him or her and with the other people in the practice and the way they do things. After all, you'll do better over the long term if you get the support you need, and your surgeon's office can be an important source of support.

So take your time in selecting the right person and practice. The information you'll find in this chapter is intended to help you to make a decision you're happy with.

Centers of Excellence

To begin, it's important that your surgeon specializes in weight-loss surgery, for a number of reasons.

First and foremost, you'll likely feel most comfortable in a practice that has a lot of experience dealing with patients in your situation. Nobody stares at someone who weighs 400 pounds in our waiting room; nobody bats an eye at the numbers that come up on the scale—unless there's something to celebrate, of course. You won't have to squeeze yourself into the chair in front of my desk when you come for your consult. And that's the way I think it should be.

There's another reason to search for someone who specializes in weight-loss surgery. The American Society for Metabolic and Bariatric Surgery found that experienced surgeons had significantly lower complication rates; the more you perform a procedure, the better you get at it, and that's true no matter what part of the body you're operating on.

I recommend that you look for a practice that has been designated a Center of Excellence. Two organizations are giving the COE designation right now—the American Society for Metabolic and Bariatric Surgery and the American College of Surgeons. These governing bodies make bariatric practices jump through a very rigorous series of hoops so that *you* can count on a certain quality of care. They send representatives to review the charts and procedures of the surgeons, the hospitals, and the staff. They also require that the surgeon enter every patient into a data bank so outcomes can be closely measured.

Among other requirements, a Center of Excellence is one that:

- has performed a large number of the procedures, and with very few complications;

- features size-appropriate furniture in both the offices and the hospitals where the procedure will be done (chairs, beds, bathroom facilities) and bariatric-appropriate medical equipment (scales, blood pressure cuffs that fit, wheelchairs that can withstand your weight, as well as bariatric surgery tools, and so on);

- has a staff trained in bariatric-specific physical and emotional issues who will be capable of providing competent and compassionate support; and

- provides appropriate and essential postoperative follow-up and care programs.

Does going with a Center of Excellence mean that you shouldn't do your own research or ask questions of your surgeon? No. All it means is that you can start out with a base level of comfort about who's doing the procedure, as well as where and how they're doing it.

There are many Centers of Excellence in the country right now, and that number grows every year, so chances are good that you're close to one.

But if you're not, or if the surgeon you've chosen isn't affiliated with one, then you may want to do a little extra legwork to reassure yourself about the standard of care. At the very least, your surgeon should be board certified in surgery and have a postoperative care program.

Not every Center of Excellence doctor is going to be perfect; likewise, there are many, many excellent surgeons who perform weight-loss surgery but are not part of a Center of Excellence because they don't get the number of cases a year to qualify. If you are far from a big city, there may not be a Center of Excellence near you, but there still may be a very good doctor.

Where to Start?

Your primary care physician (PCP) may be able to refer you to a bariatric surgeon. If you like your doctor—and the surgeon she or he refers you to—that's a good place to start.

The American Society for Metabolic and Bariatric Surgery also has a searchable database of doctors and Centers of Excellence on their Web site, ASBS.org.

Web sites such as ObesityHelp.com also feature searchable databases with thousands of doctors listed by location, complete with patient reviews.

HOME OR AWAY?

People come to see my father and me from all over the country—we've even had patients come from Europe and Asia. As flattering as that might be, in most cases, I'd suggest that you look for a local surgeon.

Keep in mind that you're going to be healing in the days immediately after the surgery, and embarking on a big trip during this time probably is not what you're going to want to be doing. You're also going to want a lot of support in the days right after—the kind you're most likely to find from friends, neighbors, and family members close to home. Being far away also means that it will be harder, if not impossible, for you to attend your surgeon's support groups, which I consider to be a really important contributor to long-term success.

On the other hand, you may need to travel, either because there's no one who does the surgeries in your immediate area or because your family and friends are somewhere else in the country, and you want to recuperate near them. When patients do travel to see me, I recommend that they 1) bring a family member or close friend who can help, and 2) stay in a hotel for at least ten days before traveling home.

If follow-up appointments aren't possible with the surgeon who did your procedure because the office is too far from home, I strongly recommend that you have your surgeon coordinate your aftercare with your PCP. And do find a support group close to you, as there's no real replacement for this experience. In a pinch, an online support group can be a good substitute; just make sure you log on!

Some people go to Mexico for surgery because it's cheaper there. This is something I discourage. You've heard the expression "you get what you pay for"? Don't get me wrong—there are some very excellent surgeons in Mexico. It will be very hard for you to determine the level of care you'll receive in advance, however, and surgery is not an area where you want to skimp on quality. And you're vulnerable, since follow-up is such a crucial part of these surgeries; most likely, you won't be able to get back to Mexico regularly, and, in my experience, most American doctors are not too excited about taking care of someone who went out of the country for the procedure.

Getting to Know the Practice

One of the great things about *Big Medicine* is that it takes a little bit of the anxiety out of that first visit; people feel like they know us and our offices already. Unless you live in Houston, you're not going to have that advantage, so you'll have to do a little sleuthing on your own. Most surgical practices have a Web site with information about the doctors, the kinds of procedures they perform, and the aftercare they provide. These sites are a good place to start.

Many weight-loss surgeons also offer seminars. A seminar is simply a presentation about weight-loss surgery, held once or twice a month. In a way, a seminar is like your first consultation. It's a time to find out more about what you can expect from surgery and for you to ask any questions you might have without any obligation. (It's also a good way to get a feel for a surgeon and his or her practice.) You might come to a seminar and decide that weight-loss surgery isn't for you; many people do. Others walk out and make their first appointment the next day.

You'll also want to make sure that your surgeon's practice offers a comprehensive bariatric program, not just the surgeries themselves.

For instance:

Psychologist. Is there a psychologist who specializes in bariatrics, and who not only evaluates patients before surgery but can offer counseling and referrals for them afterward?

Insurance support. Will the office help in dealing with your insurance company? Is there someone on staff who knows what your company requires and can help you to get your paperwork together, if not submit it on your behalf?

Dieticians. Are there registered dieticians on staff who can offer support before and after the operation? Dieticians and nutritionists are great educators. Not only can they help you to figure out what 70 grams of protein looks like, but they can also help you to isolate your particular food-related trouble spots (see the box below) and can offer ideas for how to work around them.

A dietician is particularly important because many insurance companies do require that you go on a medically supervised diet before you can be eligible for the surgery; the dietician's paperwork must be meticulous or you run the risk of rejection.

WHAT ARE YOUR FOOD BEHAVIORS?

Your dietician may ask you questions about your food behaviors and lifestyle. I think it's a good thing for everyone to answer a questionnaire like the one below.

- Do you eat breakfast, lunch, and dinner? If not, which meal do you usually skip? Do you eat these meals at roughly the same time every day?

- Is the majority of the food you eat: a) home-cooked, b) prepared at home but from a package, or c) prepared in a restaurant?

- What are your favorite foods? Do you eat them every day? Often (a few times a week)? Or do you reserve them for special occasions (once a month)?

- Do you consider yourself a "sweet" or "salty" eater?

- Do any of these foods trigger overeating or binge behavior—an inability to stop eating that food or others?

- Do you drink soda? If so, how much and how often?

- Do you drink alcohol? If so, how much and how often?

- Do you exercise? If so, how much and how often? Do you go through periods of regular exercise punctuated by periods of inactivity? If so, what causes you to stop? (pain or injury, time pressure, lack of motivation)

- Do you snack, or "graze" throughout the day? What time of day are you most likely to overeat? Do you snack in the afternoon or at night?

- Are there activities that you associate with food (watching television, going to the movies, driving, and so on)?

- Do you sometimes eat when you're not hungry? If so, why? (anxiety, stress, boredom, fatigue, depression, for comfort)

- Do you feel out of control when you are eating, as if you can't stop?

Remember: Although you will experience much less hunger after the surgery, unhealthy patterns and food behaviors can still impede your progress. Talk to someone! Your bariatric practice is there to make sure you get the help you need.

Bariatric program coordinators/nurses. Surgeons are often busy doing surgery. Is there someone on staff besides your surgeon who can answer quick questions you might have after surgery, such as what medications are appropriate to take for a headache?

Support groups. Does the office offer support groups? If so, are there different groups for different populations? (Our hospital, just to give an example, offers a general support group, a nutrition group, a fitness group, and a few smaller, more specialized support groups for patients to attend.)

Exercise help. Is there someone on staff who can offer fitness advice or refer you to a personal trainer with bariatric experience?

Special-needs assistance. You'll also want to think carefully about any special needs or requirements you have. For instance, the hospitals we work with offer translation services for patients or patients' relatives who don't speak English. Trust me, it's better than relying on my Spanish!

Questions to Ask Your Surgeon

Some people are attracted to my dad's no-nonsense, more old-fashioned doctoring style; others feel more comfortable with mine, which tends to be a little more holistic. It doesn't matter what style you prefer, but it is important that you feel comfortable with your surgeon. After all—unlike, say, knee surgery—this is a relationship that will continue long after the anesthesia has worn off.

I never mind when new patients ask questions—in fact, I prefer it. It shows me that they've done their research. Here are some of the questions I've fielded:

Are you a member of the American Society for Metabolic and Bariatric Surgery, and is the practice considered a Center of Excellence?

What percentage of your practice is bariatric medicine?

How many cases are done a year by the practice?

What are your complication and mortality rates?

What are the complications you see most often with the procedure I'm getting?

If the procedure isn't covered by insurance, do you offer financing options?

Do you do open or laparoscopic procedures? What's your "conversion to open" rate?

How long will I have to wait for surgery once I get approved?

If there's one rule I have with my patients, whether before or after surgery, it's this:

If you have a question, ask it.

Trust me, there's no question too gross or weird or trivial or off the wall to ask your doctor. That's what we're here for. I consider these interactions with my patients to be a valuable learning experience, for both them and me; in fact, they're the source of much of what you'll find in this book!

It's very common for people to forget the questions they meant to ask me once they're actually sitting in my office. To avoid this, write your questions down beforehand. Better yet, as you read this book, keep a notebook by your side so you can jot down questions as they arise.

Before you decide on a surgeon:

Go online. Read patient reviews on the Web. Web sites such as ObesityHelp.com often have reviews of surgeons. *Proceed with caution.* There isn't a doctor on the planet who doesn't have some unhappy patients—even me! And, I'm sorry to say, the unhappy ones are the ones most likely to post. On the other hand, a number of Web sites will remove negative comments about doctors for a fee, so in order to be safe, let this be one line of inquiry among many.

Talk to previous patients. Ask to attend one of the practice's support groups; this probably is the fastest way to meet people who have been operated on by your doctor. It's a great thing to do anyway—you'll learn a lot from hearing the true-life stories of people who have had these procedures. Be sure to get permission before you show up; many small surgical support groups are closed to outsiders.

||||||||||||

Once you've found a surgeon you feel comfortable with, it's time to start what some of my patients refer to as the hardest part of the whole ordeal: battling with the insurance company.

|||||||||||||||||||||||||||||||||||||||||||||||||||||||||||||||||||||||||||

CHAPTER SEVEN

Navigating the Insurance Process

A growing number of states have passed laws requiring insurance companies to provide coverage for weight-loss surgery for patients who meet the NIH guidelines. But most have not.

If you watch my show, you've seen how often my team and I have been perplexed by the decisions of the insurance companies. I will just say this: I believe that the health and well-being of the patient should play a more dominant role in the decisions of most insurance companies than they do right now.

There is hard scientific evidence that these surgeries not only increase life expectancy, but they also resolve or lessen life-threatening (and, from the insurance company's perspective, expensive) co-morbidities. In many cases, these surgeries are the only thing proven to do so. And they pay for themselves in a relatively short period of time, given the hospitalization and medication costs for co-morbidities.

It is baffling to me, then, that so many of my patients have such a difficult time convincing their insurance companies to assume responsibility. But what I think is not the issue; the goal of this chapter is to give you what you need to get your particular insurance company to say yes.

Read Your Certificate of Coverage

The first thing you need to do is read your Certificate of Coverage, or COC. This document describes your insurance policy in detail, including what it covers and what it excludes. If you don't have one, you may need to request it from the insurance company or from your human resources department at work.

WHAT IF WEIGHT-LOSS SURGERY IS NOT COVERED?

Here's what you *don't* want to see: that weight-loss surgery is excluded from your insurance coverage. But even if that's the case, don't lose heart—it's not the end of the road. Your employer determines which services and procedures the insurance they offer will cover, and it's possible to change their policy about the surgery.

One option is to get together a group of people who are interested in the surgery and present a unified front to your employer. Every year, there's more evidence that weight-loss surgery results in a better, healthier, more productive workforce.

Or you can make a personal appeal to the HR department. Include references to the science of weight-loss surgery, including journal articles showing that these surgeries are not only safe, but they are also effective at resolving obesity and many of the health conditions experienced by the obese. Share your personal story, and help the company to understand how your bariatric surgery will benefit the company as a whole, explaining that you'll have more energy and fewer health issues afterward.

If your employer does decide to cover your surgery, they have two options: They can override the policy for your particular case by buying a rider, or they can add it to the policy when they renew. (That will mean extra waiting time, but that's better than the alternative.)

Assuming that your insurance company does cover weight-loss surgery, make sure you know exactly which surgeries they cover, which expenses they cover, and whether your chosen surgeon and hospital are included in your plan. And just because they do cover the surgery doesn't mean you're approved! Check the fine print: You've got some work to do first.

Talk to Your PCP

Your insurance company may require that you be referred to a bariatric surgeon by your primary care physician. Many insurance companies require a letter of medical necessity, not just from your bariatric surgeon but also from your PCP. (You'll find a sample of a letter your family doc can write in support of your application in the Appendix on page 275.) And most companies also require medical records for a specified period before surgery demonstrating that you have been obese for at least five years.

HELP! I HAVEN'T BEEN TO A DOCTOR!

In some cases, people come to us without medical records for the previous five years. If your insurance company requires them, your best strategy is to call and see what they will accept in lieu of these records. One patient asked her psychotherapist, who had been seeing her for over five years, to write a letter on her behalf, stating that she'd been obese for the whole time she'd been his patient. Others have used dated family photographs to document their history of obesity.

Before You apply

Before your doctor submits your claim to the insurance company for preauthorization, you'll have to meet with a number of specialists, including a psychologist, a dietician, and perhaps even a sleep specialist. Most insurance companies require that you go on a medically supervised diet. The wait is annoying, but it does give you a little time to get your ducks in a row. In the land of insurance, documentation is king!

Here are some of the things you'll want to be able to document:

- How long you have been obese, including your weight and BMI every year for at least the last five years. (Many companies will require your medical records for this purpose.)

- A detailed list of medical conditions caused by your obesity.

- Every visit you have made to a health-care professional for obesity-related issues.

- A history of the medications taken to address these conditions.

- Details of the effects these conditions have had on your life. These can range from medical disability to being unable to maintain personal hygiene, trouble sleeping, or an inability to tie your own shoes. If you see any specialists, ask them to add a letter in support. For instance, if your orthopedist thinks your bad knee is a result of your extra weight, then get her or him to write a letter.

- A detailed history of your dieting efforts, complete with medical records. Receipts for diet centers, medically supervised weight-loss programs, personal trainers, and fitness club memberships are all useful. Food logs and weight journals are also useful.

You—or your surgeon's office—will use this information to prepare a letter of medical necessity in order to get your insurance company to agree to pay for your surgery. I also suggest you get letters from any other doctors that are treating you for co-morbidities from obesity. For instance, if you ave a bad knee, get a letter from your orthopedist stating that weight-loss 'gery will help your knee.

You'll find a sample of the letter we send in the Appendix on page 278. ce that we don't just establish the patient's morbid obesity but also go 'etail about obesity-related medical conditions and the effects these 'ons have had on her health and quality of life.

long will it take to find out? In general, once we've submitted the , we have an answer within thirty days, but this can vary by insur- ny. If you haven't heard anything in a month, follow up with your ce or with your insurance company.

Good to know. Get the name and extension of the person you're speaking with at the insurance company. Ask them for an e-mail address or a direct extension where they can be reached again; it will make your life easier if you can build a rapport with someone who is familiar with your case.

Appealing a Denial

If your request is denied by your insurance company, you may be able to appeal the decision. (In fact, some companies are rumored to approve only those requests that are appealed.) You can do so by writing an appeal letter. In these letters, we go through a company's criteria—one by one—and answer each of them with as much detail and documentation as we possibly can.

Options After Appeal

Even if your appeal is denied, there are still a few other options available to you. Your bariatric program will know whether you're eligible for an independent review, available to people in more than forty states, in which your insurance company will sit down with your doctor to review your specific case.

The final option is litigation—a lawsuit. Some lawyers are beginning to specialize in suits against insurance companies to get bariatric surgery covered; your surgeon's office may be able to direct you to someone who has helped their patients in the past. Again, this will be difficult—if not impossible—if your insurance company has an outright exclusion of service; if it is not a covered service, then they do not have to pay.

And, yes, there is one other option:

Paying for Surgery Yourself

If all else fails and your health insurance will not cover the surgery, you can pay for it—or for part of it—yourself.

This is a big decision, and a big financial commitment for you and your family. Bypasses cost between $20,000 and $30,000. The band is less expensive, ranging between $12,000 and $20,000—but that's still a big chunk of change!

As expensive as it is, I have quite a large number of patients who have decided that their health was worth it, and none of them would have done anything differently. If you look at the mortality statistics that begin on page 7, it's really like you're buying years of life—and who can put a price on that?

If you do decide to go it alone, talk to your surgeon's office. Most will offer some type of financing plan. Companies such as CareCredit specialize in extending credit for medical expenses, and the company that makes the band will offer a financing program to those who are interested.

If you self-pay, you may want your PCP to submit your follow-up blood work. You can end up with a big bill if these are submitted by a weight-loss surgeon.

Good to know. If you pay for your surgery yourself, there may be tax benefits. Since the IRS recognizes obesity as a disease, some of the medical expenses you incur in the treatment of that disease are deductible. Talk to your accountant about what percentage of your surgery and related expenses can be deducted from your taxes.

GOOD NEWS FOR MEDICARE PATIENTS

The government, after reviewing the evidence, has agreed that weight-loss surgery should be a covered benefit. It has stipulated, however, that Medicare will only cover the surgery if the surgeon and hospital are designated as a Center of Excellence.

CHAPTER EIGHT

Getting Ready for Surgery

"I felt like a kid waiting for Christmas when I got my surgery date."

"I was nervous, but preparation helped a lot. It felt like I was creating a little nest I could return to and heal—rather than jumping headfirst into the abyss."

I'm a big believer in preparation, and this surgery is no exception. In the months leading up to the big day, I encourage my patients to think of themselves as in training, the way they would if they were preparing for an athletic event. Surgery makes *a lot* of demands on your body: The more you can do to give your body what it needs to make it through the ordeal and toward the healing process, the better off you'll be.

The surgery is also just the beginning of what promises to be a pretty major life change. You're going to be asked to make some very significant alterations to your lifestyle in the days immediately after surgery. Unfortunately, that's not going to be your finest hour: Not only will you be recovering from major surgery, but you'll be doing so on a fraction of the calories you're consuming right now. So I recommend that you get yourself nicely set up beforehand.

**The more you have in place before surgery,
the better off you're going to be afterward.**

The point of this advice is not to scare you but to prepare you. The best-case scenario is that you step out of the operating room, right into your new life—a new life you've thought about, and planned for, in advance.

This chapter contains some of the things that I recommend my patients do in preparation for surgery. I've organized these guidelines in stages. First, I'll talk about the steps your doctor will ask you to take in order to be approved for a surgery date. Next, I'll go through what to do once you've been given that date, including what you should do the week before, the day before, and the day of.

Before You Are Given Your Surgery Date

Psychiatric Evaluation. Before we can approve you for weight-loss surgery, you need to go through a psychiatric evaluation. If you've seen the show, then you've seen our terrific psychotherapist, Mary Jo Rapini, at work.

The very thought of this evaluation puts a lot of people on edge, but it shouldn't. We're not trying to evaluate whether you're crazy—just whether or not you're emotionally ready for surgery and how you'll respond once it's over. We want to know that you're going into this process with a realistic attitude about what you can expect and what will be required of you afterward. We want to know that you'll have lots of help from your friends and family or that you have another support network in place.

The counselor can help you to identify potential trouble spots that can halt your progress after surgery and help you to come up with some ways to cope. For instance, if food is your best friend, you have to be prepared for the fact that we're about to take it away. If you're prone to depression and "medicate" yourself with food, you're going to need alternate means after surgery, whether that's through counseling or medication.

A word of advice: Don't lie! Occasionally someone tries to slip something by Mary Jo. For us, that's a much bigger red flag than candidly admitting that they've struggled with depression or addiction. Thankfully, Mary Jo is extremely experienced and doesn't miss a beat. But even if you think you can slip something by the person doing your evaluation, don't. It is far, far better to get the help you need before surgery—even if it means waiting—than to go through with the procedure and to find yourself unable to cope on the other end.

Dietary Evaluation. Your surgeon may also ask that you meet with a dietician associated with his or her office. (It's very important that this person be a specialist in obesity and have experience with weight-loss surgery, as you'll have very specific dietary needs.)

The dietician will ask you about your diet history and can help you to determine what kind of an eater you are—which may in turn help you not only to determine which surgery you should consider but also what support you may need after surgery. For instance, if you're someone with a real sweet tooth, you may want to consider the bypass, because sugars are very poorly tolerated after this surgery—they make you sick. Other people aren't tempted by dessert but have an impossible time avoiding crunchy, salty foods like chips. Knowing that these are unhealthy foods that you have not been able to enjoy in reasonable portions is an important piece of information: You'll probably need to avoid them outright after surgery.

The dietician will also explain exactly what your postsurgical diet will look like. He or she will be able to provide you with a wealth of helpful material, including sample menus, examples of portion sizes, lists of the best sources of protein, and information about artificial sweeteners. This information will be hugely important after surgery, so listen carefully, ask lots of questions, and save everything your dietician gives you.

Many insurance companies require that patients go through a medically supervised weight-loss program prior to surgery. If that's true in your case, you will be supervised by your dietician.

After You Get Your Date

Congratulations! You've got a surgery date! You're ready to take the first step in this life-changing journey.

DON'T LET IT EXPIRE!

Usually my patients want to schedule their surgeries immediately after they get insurance approval. But some people need to postpone surgery for a little while, usually because their insurance is only paying for part of it, and they need some time to get the rest of the money together. Find out when your approval expires. It's usually a fairly long time—six months or more—but it's good to make sure; you'd hate to have to go through the whole insurance process again!

Once we have a date on the calendar, these are some of the things I tell my patients to do before surgery:

Lose weight. I know—losing weight before your weight-loss surgery sounds like a bad joke. But it's no joke: Losing weight before surgery can really reduce your risk of complications. The higher your BMI, the greater the risks; as you lower your BMI, the risks come down. (This is especially true for people whose BMI is over 50.)

I generally put my patients on a protein-rich, low-carb liquid diet for at least two weeks before surgery. During this time, you drink a specially formulated weight-loss drink four to five times a day, keeping your calories under 1000 and virtually eliminating carbs. There are several benefits to a high-protein diet, including shrinking your liver (see the box below), which helps the surgery to go faster (always a good thing) and reduces bleeding.

AN ARGUMENT AGAINST THE LAST SUPPER

I certainly can understand the temptation to have one last all-you-can-eat, high-calorie, high-fat hurrah.

But here's one big reason not to: your liver.

Indulge me in a little lecture in gross anatomy. When a doctor is operating on your stomach, your liver is right there. I mean, *right there*; it actually has to be moved out of the way and held in place so we can work on your stomach. High-fat meals—even one—can swell your liver, making it bigger and harder to get out of the way, and that's dangerous, plain and simple. You do not want your surgeon struggling with your liver.

People who have been overweight for a long time often have enlarged livers; as you'll remember, nonalcoholic liver disease is a common co-morbidity of obesity. Reducing carbs is the fastest way to shrink your liver down to a healthier size, which is why I recommend that my patients follow a low-carb liquid diet in the weeks before surgery.

The other reason not to end your presurgical life with one last blowout is a psychological one. When you indulge in a last supper, what you're really saying is "This is the last time I'll ever eat normal food again." But if you take a minute to think about that message, you'll see why it's fundamentally wrong. First of all, no matter what surgery you're having, you'll be eating "real," "normal" foods again in a matter of weeks. And the point of this surgery is to get out of the "on a diet, off a diet" mind-set. This is a change you're making for the rest of your life—and, for best results, your commitment to that change needs to begin right now.

Exercise. The more you exercise before surgery, the easier the surgery will go. Exercise improves circulation—and as you already know, blood clots are one of the risks of these surgeries, particularly in the very obese. Exercise also increases your lung capacity.

Exercise also speeds recovery. You'll be walking as soon as you wake up from the anesthesia, and I give my patients a series of exercises that I like them to do to help in their recovery. Do these every day as soon as your surgeon gives them to you: It'll be much easier for you if you aren't learning them for the first time on the other end.

If you don't do any exercise, then just go for a walk and try to increase the distance and speed every day before your operation. It will make a huge impact on your ability to withstand the stress of the operation. Beginning an exercise routine now also means that you won't have to begin one afterward; you'll just be picking up where you left off. And, finally, exercise can be a healthy way for you to discharge some of the anxiety you might be feeling about the approaching changes.

Keep your skin in good shape. A skin breakdown can lead to an infection—and to a postponement of your surgery. If you're prone to skin breakdowns, make sure to shower at least once every day using an antibacterial surgical soap. Make sure to keep infection-prone areas as dry as possible by using a hair dryer on low heat after your shower followed by a sprinkling of cornstarch. (If you use baby powder, put your underwear on first before applying: too much exposure can lead to urinary tract infections.)

If you're prone to skin breakdown due to friction, try a protective barrier. Some of my patients swear by roll-on deodorant liberally applied to areas that tend to get damp; do a patch test on the inside of your elbow to see if that's a good solution for you. A number of athletic companies also make roll-on gels, such as BodyGlide, which are designed to reduce skin friction.

Check your medications. Before surgery, your doctor should know *exactly* what medications you take and what's in them.

Just because it's over the counter doesn't mean it's safe before surgery! Aspirin and medications that contain aspirin should be discontinued at least ten days before surgery, for instance, because they are blood thinners. (Tylenol is still okay if you find yourself with a headache or muscle pain.)

And don't forget about the stuff you got at the health food store, either. St. John's wort, ginkgo biloba, and garlic are examples of natural supplements that also should be discontinued. Some herbal supplements, such as kava and valerian, have been shown to interfere with anesthetics.

You'll also want to ask which of your daily medications are okay to take the day of surgery—some can be taken with a small sip of water; others we'll ask you to skip—and which ones you'll be discontinuing after surgery.

If any other doctors prescribe you meds, let them know you will not be able to take extended-release tablets or large-size tablets or capsules after surgery. If you are on extended-release medications, you should get those changed preoperatively. Some surgeons also will discontinue diuretics, so let your family doc know. If you are diabetic, you will likely leave the hospital on a sliding scale of insulin. This should be set up prior to surgery and you should have all necessary supplies, including needles, syringes, and blood sugar monitor.

Take a multivitamin. A multivitamin is a general health booster and a good idea for everyone. It is amazing to me how many people have vitamin deficiencies before surgery.

Important: Check your multivitamin! Herbal supplements are making their way into more and more multivitamins, and some of these ingredients could put you at risk during surgery. Make sure your surgeon knows exactly what's in yours.

Quit smoking. I won't operate on a smoker, and none of the surgeons I know will. Why? Smoking interferes with lung function, increasing the possibility of anesthetic complications. Not to mention that blood clots are a major risk during this surgery, and one that is unacceptably exacerbated by smoking. Smoking can also slow healing. And if you're having a bypass, smoking after surgery will lead you right to an ulcer.

My patients are required to stop smoking at least six weeks before surgery. Seize this opportunity; it's just another way that weight-loss surgery will improve your health for the better.

Eat lots of protein. Protein is what your body needs to heal. If you're not on a high-protein liquid diet in preparation for the surgery, at least make sure to include lots of lean, high-protein meats, such as chicken and turkey, low-fat dairy, such as skim milk and yogurt, as well as beans and nuts into your diet.

Drink lots of fluids and get lots of rest. Stay hydrated.

If you have a cold, fever, respiratory infection, or any other infection, including one in your teeth, the week before surgery, let your doctor know.

The Week Before Surgery

Your goal this week is to clear the decks as much as possible so that postsurgery you can focus your energy on recuperating—and to make sure you'll have everything you need when you get home.

Call the hospital. Having a few questions answered will make your stay much more pleasant. Will there be a phone in your room? If not, is there a public phone on the floor? (Cell phones are prohibited in most hospitals, so you'll want to show up with your address book. And if there's no phone in your room, or if you'll want to call long distance, you'll need plenty of quarters or a calling card.)

Find out when visiting hours are so you can tell friends and family before the procedure. If you have any other special needs—spiritual or translation services, for instance—ask about them now.

Set up your house. Make sure your house is well set up to accommodate you after the operation. Some ideas:

Do laundry, and leave it out where it'll be easily accessible.

Figure out how you're going to get in and out of the shower and on and off the toilet in the days immediately after surgery. A bariatric-appropriate toilet seat lift and shower chair, available for rent at surgical supply stores, are a couple of things you may want to consider.

Stop drinking caffeinated and carbonated beverages. Caffeine is a diuretic, and after surgery we don't want you to get dehydrated, so you must avoid caffeine, at least in the beginning. Quit ahead of time and you won't have to deal with withdrawal symptoms—headaches, crankiness—after your surgery. Get it over with now!

Stock up on entertainment. You're not going to be hitting the town for a little while after you get home. Buy books, magazines, and puzzles, and borrow some DVDs to enjoy during your recovery.

Tie up loose ends. If you're going to need any other special items at home before surgery, this is a good time to pick them up. It's also a good time to refill medications (ask your surgeon first!), to pay bills, and to check other essentials off the to-do list. Make sure you've made adequate childcare and pet-care plans for your time in the hospital and the recuperation. Will it be a problem if you need to stay in the hospital an extra night or two?

Out with the old, in with the new. You don't want to come home to a kitchen that's loaded with all the foods that got you here in the first place. This is a great time to take a big trash bag and get rid of all the unhealthy foods you find in your cupboards. (Your spouse and kids don't need them either—trust me.)

That doesn't mean leaving your larder bare. After you've finished your cleanout, go grocery shopping for the staple items you'll want to have around after surgery (see page 107 for a shopping list).

This is also a good time to make and freeze batches of some of your

YOUR PRESURGICAL GROCERY LIST

Go shopping and have these things waiting for you at home so planning and making your post-op meals goes smoothly.

Note: You probably won't be able to eat all of these foods in the first few weeks after your surgery, but they're good to have on hand; you'll move fairly quickly into the next phase.

Food and Drink

Fat-free broths, clear soups, and bouillion cubes (beef, chicken, and vegetable)

Unsweetened clear juice (you'll limit this to one cup a day after surgery)

Skim, soy, or 1% milk (some people don't tolerate milk well after surgery, but you can try)

Eggs

Cream of wheat or other completely smooth, whole-grain cereal

No-sugar-added Carnation Instant Breakfast

No-sugar-added fruit pops (with no fruit chunks)

Sugar-free yogurt (I like Greek-style yogurts like FAGE Total; they're also higher in protein)

Protein powder

Protein shakes (like Isopure zero carb)

Frozen fruits (plain, not sweetened or in syrup)

Soft tofu

Fat-free or low-fat cottage cheese

Herbal teas, decaf coffee
Artificial sweetener (Splenda)
Agave nectar (a low-glycemic sweetener)

Supplements

Multivitamins
Gas-X or something similar

If you're having a bypass, you'll also need:

Sublingual vitamin B_{12}
Iron
Calcium citrate with vitamin D
Tylenol in liquid form (After your bypass, you won't be able to take anti-inflammatories such as Advil for headache or muscle pain anymore—and liquid medications will be easiest for you to tolerate while your pouch is still swollen.)

Supplements should be chewable. For more information on what kind of supplements to look for, see page 153.

Wound-Care Supplies

You may also want to pick up some wound-care supplies, including gauze pads, bandage tape, cotton balls, hydrogen peroxide, and a heating pad for the days immediately after surgery. You should also purchase a thermometer if you don't have one.

Gear

Measuring cups. It can be very helpful, especially in the first few weeks after surgery, to measure your food. Your new portion sizes will be drastically reduced, and it might take you a little time to get adept at estimating them. Measuring can prevent accidental overeating, which can be quite painful!

Food scale. Again, a food scale can be very helpful in helping you to understand how much food your new stomach can tolerate.

Baby spoons. Using small spoons, such as the ones designed for toddlers (found in the baby aisle at most drugstores) is a good way to remind yourself to slow down and take small bites. One of my patients uses the decorated teaspoons she's collected from all over the world; another uses the smallest spoons from her grandmother's silver service.

Small containers. Again, this is something that might help with portion control, and it's nice to have an appropriate-size container so your meal doesn't look so lost! Back to the baby aisle: Many of my patients use the small containers with lids that you can find there.

Ice cube trays. As I mentioned earlier, these are invaluable for freezing appropriate-size portions of homemade foods. Some people also freeze unsweetened fruit juice into cubes. These juice cubes add a little zip to a big glass of plain water, without the calories and sugar of straight juice.

Snack-size zip-top bags. These are roughly half the size of a traditional sandwich-size bag and can help with appropriate portioning; they're great for when you're on the go. If you buy a large container of a food that you find hard to portion control, you can also use these small-size zip-top bags to break them down into 100-calorie snack packs when you get home from the grocery store.

Utensils and containers for eating and drinking on the go. You're probably going to find that "bringing your own" is the best option a lot of the time; not having the supplies you need shouldn't be an excuse! Depending on where you're likely to be eating, some options you may want to consider include plastic or bamboo disposable flatware, paper bags, a hot/cold thermos, or a small cooler.

One of my patients went to a Japanese specialty store and bought children's bento boxes for everyone in her support group. Get creative!

Hygiene

Abdominal surgery means that you're likely to have some difficulty maneuvering in the bathroom after the surgery. You may want to pick up some things to help in advance of the procedure:

Flushable wipes

Peri Bottle (available at medical supply stores; a sports-top water bottle will work just as well)

Long-handled sponge stick

favorite foods, as long as they're low-calorie and low-fat and will be appropriate after surgery. If you preportion before you freeze, remember your new portion sizes! Many of my patients use ice cube trays; that way they can snap out two or three "cubes" of their favorite soups or puréed meals, pop them into a microwave, and—voilà—dinner!

Arrange for time off work. With the band, you may go home the same day after surgery. You'll be up and walking and active immediately. I usually tell my patients they can return to work in one to two weeks, although you really should not do any lifting (of anything that weighs more than thirty pounds) for at least a month.

I keep my patients in the hospital for two nights after bypass, although some surgeons require only one night. Bypass patients are usually up and about in a week or two also (we use the same small incisions with the bypass as we do with the band), but bypass patients usually take two to three weeks off work. They're losing weight more quickly and can feel a little more fatigued.

Of course, some people bounce back from surgery right away and are raring to go in a week; others find the first month after surgery to be physically and emotionally overwhelming. I advise my patients to take as much time as they possibly can, especially if their job has a physical component.

TO TELL OR NOT TO TELL?

My patients often ask me whether or not they should tell their colleagues at work that they're having weight-loss surgery.

The answer, of course, is different for everyone. In truth, it's nobody's business but your own, but talking about it does tend to make the aftermath easier. You won't have to explain the small portions and the amazing shrinking body, and given that most of us spend as much—or more!—time with the people at work than we do with our family and friends, our work friends can be another important potential source of support.

Even if you choose to keep the details private, it's important that the people in your workplace know that you are recovering from pretty major abdominal surgery and won't be able to lift or carry anything for a while.

If your work needs you (or you need the paycheck!) sooner rather than later, see if there are some accommodations you can make for the later weeks, like going in for half the day or catching up on some things from home.

Remember that we do not want you driving for at least one week, or until you have absolutely no pain at all. So you may have to carpool or be dropped off.

Enlist or hire a caregiver. How much help you need, and for how long, will depend mostly on your physical condition; your doctor's office will be able to help you determine a realistic estimate. But even the most fit and independent patient will benefit from having someone around to help for the first week or so.

You'll need someone to come to the hospital with you and to be there after surgery. You'll also need someone to take you home from the hospital, and I recommend having someone stay with you for the first week as well. If your family members can't accommodate or will be gone for long stretches, you may want to arrange for a friend or neighbor to stop by.

If no friend or relative can come and stay with you for a little while, or if you'll need extra help after surgery because of other medical illnesses or another reason, talk to your doctor about the possibility of an extended-care facility or part-time in-home help.

Meet with your surgeon. You'll be scheduled for an appointment about a week before your surgery. You'll talk to your surgeon (this is a good time to raise any last-minute questions or concerns) and sign your surgical consent form. We'll also order some presurgical tests. Which tests you receive depends on your personal medical history.

These are some of the tests your surgeon may order:

- *H. pylori:* This gastrointestinal bacteria raises the likelihood of ulcers after a bypass. We ask you to breathe into a machine to determine if you have it (it's symptomless, so you could have it without knowing); if you do, we'll put you on antibiotics to get rid of it.

- Blood count

- Urinalysis

- Chest X-ray

- Coagulation studies

- Test for anemia

- Liver function test

- Stress test and heart workup

- EGD: If you have reflux, we may look at your esophagus and stomach with a scope to make sure there aren't any ulcers.

- Sleep study: If you snore or find yourself tired during the day, we may order a sleep study to determine whether or not you have sleep apnea, a condition that can be extremely dangerous in combination with narcotics.

At this appointment your surgeon will give you pre-op instructions. You'll also get the lowdown on the preadmission policy at the hospital (each hospital has its own set of procedures and requirements for admitting patients), and you'll make an appointment for your first follow-up visit.

The Day Before Surgery

Go for a walk in the morning; it's good to get your circulation going before surgery.

Pack your bag. You won't be in the hospital for long—I often send band patients home the same day; even my bypass patients sometimes feel ready to leave after one night in the hospital—so you won't need a lot.

I usually tell my patients to bring:

- A robe and some nonslip slippers (remember, you're going to be walking right away).

- Basic toiletries: a toothbrush and toothpaste, deodorant, hand lotion, a hairbrush, and some lip balm.

- Your medications, CPAP (Continuous positive airway pressure) machine if you use one, and reading glasses and a contact lens care kit if you need it.

- Your favorite pillow—some people feel better if they have their own pillow, and I often see a small framed picture of a child or a pet by the bed when I do my rounds. If there's something small (nothing valuable or irreplaceable, please!) that will make you feel more at home, bring it along.

- A couple of light magazines—they can help you while away the time if you're going to be staying overnight (you may have some difficulty concentrating on anything more substantial after the anesthesia).

- A small amount of money—don't bring more than $20 for forgotten toiletries and sundries, and leave valuables like jewelry and laptops at home.

You're going to spend the rest of the day before surgery relaxing close to home. Here's why:

Bowel preparation. Since this is surgery on the stomach and intestines, some bowel preparation is necessary. (Some surgeons will require that you do a bowel prep before a bypass but not a band.)

The day before surgery, you'll drink only clear liquids, including water, tea, apple, grape, and cranberry juices, broth, and clear (not fudge) ice pops. You may be asked to take something to clean you out early in the day—my patients take magnesium citrate.

The Night Before Surgery

Take care of yourself. Remove your toenail- and fingernail polish; you will have an oxygen saturation monitor attached to one of your fingers, which uses the color of your nail to read the level of oxygen in your blood.

You can, of course, shower the morning of, but if your surgery time is very early, you may want to get it out of the way the night before. It's a good idea to use a surgical soap such as Hibiclens in the shower. And here's a little insider tip: the OR nurses are going to use a cotton swab to clean out your navel, and they consider it a tremendous courtesy if you've taken a pass at it first. Prepare to leave all jewelry and other valuables at home. (Your wedding ring can be taped if it won't come off your finger.)

Don't have anything to eat or drink after midnight. No breath mints or chewing gum, either.

Finally, get lots of sleep—you've got a big day ahead of you!

CHAPTER NINE

||||||||||||||||||||||||||||||||||||||||||||||||||||||||||

The Big Day

On your surgery day, very little is actually required of you.

Before you leave home

Shower (if you didn't last night). Don't apply makeup, perfume, body cream, or face lotion. Wear comfy, loose-fitting clothes, and pack another set to come home in. (You'll want lots of room in the abdominal area in particular.)

Don't wear your contact lenses. Remember to bring cases for your glasses, your dentures, and your hearing aid.

If you'll need any medications, such as insulin or an inhaler, bring them with you. Take your daily medication, as long as your surgeon told you it was okay.

Be on time. I ask my patients to be there two hours before surgery. (We can't set up instruments until you're in the hospital.) I'll want to say hi, and your anesthesiologist will see you before the surgery; we'll also start an IV line to give you liquids and medications if you need them.

Take a picture! If you're a scrapbook type—or even if you're not—you'll appreciate this last shot of the "old" you. Many of my patients document their weight loss in pictures; it can be a very inspirational record, and a shot taken just outside the hospital on the morning of surgery is often the first entry.

Sign a consent form. You already may have done this at your doctor's office, but you're also legally required to do it again right before surgery. The consent form will list the surgeon, the procedure, and all the risks of surgery. It can be scary to read, but no scarier than the package insert for your average over-the-counter pain medication.

Be prepared for people to ask you over and over—and over and over—which surgery you are having. This is a checklist process and nothing to worry about, but I understand that it can be unnerving when every person you meet asks as if they didn't know.

I'M SCARED!

It's pretty natural to be scared; even routine surgery is a big deal, and hospitals give lots of people the heebie-jeebies.

Preparation helps. Look hard and wide for the best surgeon in your area, and ask all the questions you can possibly think of before. In my experience, the best-prepared patients are the ones raring to hit the operating room—and the new life waiting for them on the other side. Remember, too, that you can significantly lower your risk by losing as much weight as possible before the surgery and by following a high-protein, low-carb diet in order to shrink your liver.

In general, I find that my most fearful patients benefit from hearing how infrequently serious problems arise. And if you're someone who's afraid to "go under," it's important to know that anesthesia is much less risky than it used to be. The monitors we use now are much more sensitive, and they can alert us to changes in your condition long before they become real problems.

You usually can have someone with you all the way up to the point when we take you into the OR. If you're feeling anxious, make sure the person with you is having a calming effect; sometimes I see spouses and family members who are far more worried than the patients! If that's the case—and if they're unwittingly making your nerves worse—it's okay to tell them that you'd like to be alone for a minute to prepare yourself for surgery. Breathe deeply, and focus on what your life will be like when you wake up.

What Happens Now?

You won't be in the OR long; I usually estimate an hour for the band and two for the bypass, although it can go much more quickly than that. (Revisions, which tend to be more complicated surgeries, can take a little longer.) This can vary by surgeon, so I would get an idea beforehand. And remember to tack on time for the OR prep. The surgery may take an hour, but your family may not see me for two hours, due to the preparation before surgery. Tell your family that they shouldn't worry if you're in there longer than planned—sometimes delays are unavoidable, and they certainly shouldn't draw any conclusions from it.

After your surgery, you'll be moved to the recovery room, where you'll wake up. Congratulations, and welcome to the losing side! You'll probably be quite woozy—but hopefully not too uncomfortable. Your throat may be sore from the tube that was there, and you may feel very thirsty.

Thankfully, there isn't a great deal of pain associated with the period after surgery. You may experience some pain around your incisions. It's certainly not uncommon for people to feel a little nausea, lightheadedness, weakness, gas pains, or a stomach ache—although many people feel none of these things.

You also may feel emotionally shaky, or positively euphoric—again, that's perfectly normal after surgery. As long as you don't agree to get engaged or divorced while you're in there, you're probably okay.

Don't suffer in silence; if you're uncomfortable in any way, tell the nurses what's going on with you, both in the recovery room and later, when you're moved to your room. (Be nice. Nurses are chronically overworked.) There are medications we can give you for pain and nausea, and it might help you to talk to someone about whatever emotional distress you're having. Everybody—your surgeon, the nursing staff, as well as your family and friends—wants you to be comfortable and happy, so communicate clearly about what would help you to move in that direction.

You may have what's called a PCA pump, which will allow you to get pain medicine by pushing a button. After you're taken off that machine, the nurses will give you liquid pain medication if you require it.

Some surgeons will have a urinary catheter inserted while you are asleep, and you will keep this overnight.

Out of bed! The single best preventative measure we can take against blood clots is to get you moving. As soon as you can, a nurse will help you to sit up or stand by your bedside. (Don't go it alone the first time, even if you feel pretty confident; your body's gone through a lot.) Getting out of bed the first time probably is not going to be the most comfortable thing in the world, but it will get easier.

You'll be encouraged to go for a short, supported walk as soon as you possibly can, and for a five-minute walk every two hours for the duration of your stay. Your doctor also will have you wear pressure stockings in the days following surgery, which will help to prevent blood clots, and the nurse may come by with a shot containing blood thinners.

In between, you'll do the following breathing and leg exercises at least once an hour, every hour.

Breathing exercises.

Inhale as deeply as you can, into the very bottom of your lungs.
Hold your breath for two full seconds.
Exhale completely.
Do this three times.
The next step is to cough—from your belly, not from your throat. A pillow held across your abdomen may help.

(The nurses may also give you a machine called an incentive spirometer. You suck on a mouthpiece, which makes a ball rise in a canister. The game is to see how high and how long you can get the ball to stay up. This has the same effect of the above exercises.)

Leg exercises. Push the toes of both feet toward the end of the bed, like you're pressing the accelerator in your car. Then flex your feet, so that your toes are pointing back toward your head. Do this between five and ten times.

Circle your ankles, in both directions, a minimum of five times.

Aside from your walking, leg, and breathing exercises, take advantage of the fact that nobody wants or needs you to do anything at all. This is a time to rest and relax.

IF YOU'RE NOT AMBULATORY

If you weren't mobile before the surgery, you won't be mobile after it—or not yet, anyway. But that doesn't mean that you shouldn't move around.

You can sit in a chair or at the end of your bed and make a walking motion, lifting each leg off the ground, returning it, and lifting the next one. If that's too much, simply push one foot away from you, sliding it across the floor, bring it back, and do the same with the other one. Do this for at least five minutes.

If nothing else, sit and dangle your legs off the edge of the bed for as long as you can. Change your position frequently. It may seem like I'm asking a lot—particularly at this time—but it really is the best thing for you.

Tests. Some doctors, me included, will have you drink a dye solution while having an X-ray taken while you're still in the hospital. This baseline study will check for any leaks from the bypass; in band patients, it ensures that everything is in the right position. Be prepared: The dye causes diarrhea later on.

Food. You probably won't be very hungry—most patients report a very limited appetite in the hospital after surgery and often for a while afterward.

It's essential to stay hydrated, so be sure to sip small amounts of water or other liquids throughout your time in the hospital, even if you don't want to—it's very easy to fall behind on this because the pouch is so swollen at this stage. We like both our band and our bypass patients to try taking 2 to 3 ounces of liquid every hour in the beginning. You'll be offered a choice of liquids, including broth and juice, a few times a day; save the glasses on your bedside table so that you can sip throughout the day. Once you get home, you should start to add protein shakes to your repertoire.

Drains. During a bypass, some surgeons will leave in a drain that comes out of your belly and ends in a small ball that applies suction to the wound. This is to protect you if there were to be a leak, and to alert the surgeon. Because the leak rate is so low now, not many surgeons use them. If you have a drain, it will put out a fluid that looks like Kool-Aid; that's what it's supposed to look like.

Usually the drain will be removed before you leave the hospital, although occasionally the surgeon may ask you to go home with it. The surgeon will give you care instructions before you leave, and he or she will pull the drain in the office. It may feel funny as it is removed, but most patients say it does not hurt very much.

Gas. It is very common to feel very bloated after surgery because we blow gas into your belly when we do laparoscopic surgery. This may even make your shoulders ache, but it should pass quickly.

Wounds. Surgeons have many different ways of bandaging wounds. I just use skin glue; others use actual bandages. I let my patients shower the next day, but other doctors—my father, for instance—will ask you not to get the incisions wet for a week. It's not a right or wrong situation but a difference of opinion, although I will say that my patients tend to smell better at their one-week visit than my father's do.

Being monitored. Sometimes you will have a heart monitor on after surgery. You will also likely get some blood drawn for tests. We just want to make sure that there's no drop in your blood counts, fast heart rates, fevers, or signs of infection. We will not release you until we feel it is safe. Doctors tend to be conservative, and if there is any question about your condition, we may keep you longer in the hospital—and if we are worried about something, we will let you know.

If we're really worried, we may suggest going back into surgery, just to take a look with a scope to be sure everything is okay—or to fix the problem, if there is one. It has been a very long while since I have done this, but it can happen.

I know this induces a great deal of worry, but do try hard to trust in the fact that you have found an excellent doctor who cares for you like he or she would care for a family member.

Open surgery. If you had open surgery, you may be staying in the hospital longer, and you will likely have more pain. Your recovery will also be slower, so modify your expectations accordingly.

Going Home

After one or two days, you'll be leaving the hospital and going back home, to your new life. Arrange for someone to drive you home. Before you leave, make sure you understand your surgeon's instructions for wound care, and confirm that you have a one- (or two-) week follow-up appointment scheduled.

Make sure you understand what medications you're supposed to continue when you get home; I often send patients home without their diabetes medications, for instance. Your doctor probably will tell you to resume taking your birth control pills (but use backup!—see page 129), thyroid medication, and any psychiatric medications when you get home. You will need different formulations, though; as we discussed on page 104, you won't be able to take extended-release medications or large pills.

If your trip home from the hospital will take more than half an hour, you're going to have to stop the car to walk around for five minutes every half hour to minimize the risk of clots.

CHAPTER TEN

||||||||||||||||||||||||||||||||||||||||||||||||||||||

Life After Surgery

The First Six Weeks

The first six weeks after surgery is a big time. Not only are you recovering from the trauma of surgery, but you're doing so on fewer calories than you're used to. You probably were eating somewhere between 3000 and 4000 calories a day before your operation—and now you're eating under 1000. That's a serious adjustment to make.

Here's what you can expect during this time, and some tips and tricks to ease you through the transition. As you'll see, I've left one (big) thing out: what you'll be eating. Don't worry—there *is* food in your future. But because diet after surgery is such a major topic, and because it will be changing quite a bit at various stages in these six weeks, I'll devote the whole next chapter to it.

·THE MOST IMPORTANT THING YOU'LL READ IN THIS CHAPTER

Follow your surgeon's postoperative instructions to the letter!

The First Week

The first week tends to be the hardest. You're not only spending a lot of energy on healing, but you're working hard to establish new habits. You may also be dealing with some pretty heavy-duty emotional stuff: sadness about the types of food and food behaviors you've left behind, nervousness that you won't be able to see this through, and fear about what comes next. You'll probably be a little sore from the surgery, and your new tummy may not be entirely cooperative.

This is a time to take it easy. Take the time to recover, and try not to rush back into "real life."

Please note: Relaxing doesn't mean taking to your bed! You'll be walking for exercise (more on that later) as soon as you get home. I also recommend that, after the first day or so, my patients take over the preparation of their own meals. It gives them an excuse to be up and about, and I think it's beneficial for you to be actively involved in the planning and execution of your new diet as soon as possible.

**The more you move,
the better you're going to feel.**

Dizziness, nausea, lack of energy, and digestive problems—constipation, loose stools, gas, maybe even vomiting—are the most common complaints. A lot of people report feeling weak and pretty exhausted; you may feel like it's taking you a long time to do the simplest thing, or that you're completely depleted by the most routine task. Don't worry: As rotten as it might feel, this period doesn't last long.

As far as food goes, you probably won't be all that interested in anything edible during this first week. In any case, to allow your stomach to heal, you'll be sticking to liquids such as broths and protein shakes.

Drink water! You may not be hungry, but you must remember to drink—often—in order to get your 48 to 64 ounces a day. If you've had a bypass, your pouch only holds 1 to 2 ounces right now, so this will be relatively hard to do; in order to make sure that you get what you need, sip a little bit *every fifteen minutes*, and keep a bottle of water with you *at all times*.

Your body will tell you if you're not drinking enough. Your urine will be dark yellow and strong smelling, and you may not urinate very often. You may also experience constipation or feel light-headed when you stand up. These are all signs of dehydration.

Pay attention to signs that your body isn't getting enough fluids, and increase your water intake accordingly.

If you're having problems taking in enough water, ice chips and sugar-free ice pops can help. Avoid juice and other calorie-loaded liquids, or keep your juice consumption to no more than a cup a day. Not only will they slow your weight loss, but fruit juice is rich in sugar, and if you've had a bypass, sugar-rich foods can cause dumping.

Coping with nausea. Nausea is one of the most common complaints we hear about. You may find that you're very sensitive to odors in the days after surgery. (Female patients often comment that it's very similar to the way they felt when they were pregnant, and they're right: There's a hormonal component to the nausea after bariatric surgery as well.)

Refrain from wearing perfumes and lotions—and ask family members to do the same. Stay away from cooking odors and poorly ventilated spaces.

Peppermint has been used for thousands of years as an antiemetic; sipping on some mint tea or sniffing a few drops of peppermint oil from a handkerchief can help. Ginger tea is also a fantastic antinausea remedy. Mix 2 teaspoons of powdered ginger (available at the grocery store) into 8 ounces of hot water, and sip.

If you believe that your pain medication is causing your nausea, call your surgeon; there are other medications you can try. If your nausea is very bad, ask about an antinausea medication.

Please note: Nausea and occasional vomiting are par for the course, but constant and repeated vomiting is abnormal. If this is happening, notify your surgeon.

Take care of your incisions. Again, surgeons have different thoughts on this. I don't mind if you get your incision and tube sites wet; in my book, showering is not just okay; it's recommended, and you can clean the sites gently with soap and water while you're in there (don't scrub!). Keep the sites clean and dry the rest of the time; pat the areas dry with a towel after you get out of your shower, and leave them uncovered unless they're catching on your clothes, in which case you can use a light dressing. You don't need to put any creams or salves on them afterward. Don't take a bath until you've gotten the green light from your surgeon.

The area probably will be quite bruised and swollen; that's normal. Wounds can also leak a little bit of bloody fluid from time to time, and that is okay. If the wound is getting bright red and blanches to the touch or is leaking a thick white/yellow/brown fluid, then notify your surgeon because you may need to start an antibiotic. Very occasionally the wound may need to be opened to allow it to drain. Sometimes you may have to do dressing changes at home. Don't worry if this happens; it will heal with time.

The area will itch as it heals, and it may also feel numb to the touch, the result of small nerves that have been cut. The sensation to those areas usually returns in a few months—you may feel small shooting electrical sensations, like little zaps, as that happens. In the meantime, be sensitive if you're using ice or heat on the area.

As your scars heal they will turn some impressive colors: red, pink, and purple are all normal. Moisturizers, especially those that contain vitamin E oil, will promote healing. Only after about two weeks, when your incisions are on the way to becoming fully healed, may you start using silicone pads and scar-minimizing creams.

Do protect your scars from the sun in the year after surgery, and remember that the sun's harmful rays can penetrate a bathing suit. Wear a minimum of SPF 15 when outside in the sun.

Thrush/yeast infections. Don't be alarmed if you notice a white, cottage cheese–like coating on your tongue, or if your tongue seems red and inflamed. This probably is thrush, which is an overgrowth of yeast in your mouth, a common side effect of the antibiotics we use to make sure you don't get an infection after surgery. Call your surgeon or your PCP if you notice these signs; a course of "good" bacteria, *Lactobacillus acidophilus*, should clear it up.

Women may also notice symptoms of a vaginal yeast infection—an uncomfortable itching and burning in the genital area, sometimes accompanied by a whitish discharge. Call your PCP or OB/GYN if you have these symptoms; they can be very effectively treated with over-the-counter medications, but more serious infections should be ruled out first. If you are prone to yeast infections, ask your doctor about taking *Lactobacillus acidophilus* along with your other medications after surgery. Wearing cotton underwear, refraining from using feminine hygiene sprays and douching, and, once you're up and about, avoiding wearing pantyhose every day may also help.

Follow-up visits. If you don't have one scheduled, make a follow-up appointment with your doctor as soon as you get home.

It varies from surgeon to surgeon, but I have my bypass patients come in for the first time about seven to ten days after surgery, and then at ever-increasing intervals: one to two months, six months, nine months, twelve months, and then yearly. (Your surgeon's schedule may be slightly different.)

Band patients will see their doctors more often for fills. Usually the band patient will come in for a checkup at seven to ten days, and then return for a fill at six weeks. Most doctors will then do monthly fills until you are in the green zone (see page 185). After that, band patients come in as they need to—but at least one time a year.

Your doctor will likely have a physician's assistant or a nurse who will be available to answer questions in between visits.

CALL YOUR DOCTOR

You'll probably experience some slight discomfort in the weeks immediately after surgery. But you should get in touch with your surgeon's office *immediately* if you have any of the following symptoms in the early days after surgery:

- Fever over 101. If you have a sustained temperature in the 100s, notify your surgeon.

- Chills

- Vomiting or serious nausea (a little is to be expected)

- Severe swelling or bruising (a little is to be expected)

- Severe pain that isn't relieved by pain medication

- Pain or swelling in your lower extremities (feet or legs)

- Pain in your abdomen above and beyond what you would normally expect

- Bright redness or discharge at the wound site

- Blood in your urine or your stool, or if it hurts to urinate. You may see blood in your stool right after your bypass, but if it continues by the time you're at home, tell your surgeon.

- Chest pain or shortness of breath

- Watch out for the signs of dehydration. If you're vomiting a lot, have diarrhea for more than two days, a dry mouth, dark urine, and/or you feel dizzy when you stand, then you may need to see your doctor.

A hernia is something else to watch out for. It will show up a few months after surgery as a bulge under the skin of your incision. (That bulge is your bowel, which is no longer contained because of a weakness in the abdominal wall around the site of your incision.) Symptoms of hernia include pain when you lift an object or cough or a sensation of strain while you're using the toilet. You may experience a dull ache that gets worse toward the end of the day or after you've been standing for a long period of time. You can minimize the risk of hernia by avoiding heavy lifting for two months after surgery, but if you suspect that you have a hernia, call your surgeon immediately. Hernias are very rare after laparoscopic surgery, but if one does occur, surgery will be required to repair it.

I tell my patients to get in touch sooner rather than later with any questions or concerns they might have after their operations. I'd much rather field a question than be called to the emergency room!

Two to Six Weeks

Most people are back on their feet and feeling great after two or three weeks. You can drive as soon as you're off pain meds and feel well enough to do it.

It takes a little longer for some people to start feeling better. (Without beating a dead horse here, I have noticed that the people who got in shape for their surgery are the ones that bounce back the quickest.) But in general, six weeks seems to be a turning point for everyone.

Fertility. You can start to have sex as soon as you feel like it, as long as you and your partner are careful of those incisions.

A word of caution: Because we may have you stop oral birth control for a little while after surgery (it can predispose you to blood clots) and because absorption of meds can be impaired initially, I recommend you use other forms of contraception in addition to the oral contraceptive for the first few months.

It's not unusual for my obese patients to laugh when I ask what they use for birth control: "We haven't used anything in years; I'm infertile, remember?" Well, infertility—in both sexes—is one of the co-morbidities that's commonly resolved or improved with these surgeries. So if you're interested in avoiding a pregnancy, you'll probably want to begin using birth control, no matter what your fertility status was before surgery.

A word about pregnancy: Most doctors will tell you to avoid getting pregnant for the first year or two after surgery. We do not want you losing weight while you are pregnant, and we need to make sure you're getting an adequate amount of nutrition to support a healthy pregnancy. With the band, we can just pull out the fluid.

So it's best to wait until you've reached your goal weight, but if you become pregnant before that, don't worry. Go to your OB/GYN as soon as possible, and ask her or him to contact your surgeon so they can collaborate together on the best possible care for you.

Start a food journal. Probably the most important habit you'll put into place in these early days is keeping a food journal. (Ideally you'll start right after surgery, but it's essential when you resume eating solid foods.)

The format is simple. You'll write down what you ate, how much, and at what time. I also recommend adding an emotional component to this by journaling how you felt before and after you ate the food.

Your journal might, look something like this:

Food Journal

	Breakfast	Lunch	Dinner	Snacks
Time				
How I Felt Before I Ate				
How I Felt After I Ate				

Here's why a food journal is so important: First of all, as I've already mentioned, studies show that we routinely consume many more calories—50 to 100 percent more—than we think we're consuming. Having patients keep a food journal is the only way I know to make sure that they stay mindful of what goes in their mouths—that they don't eat an entire meal's worth of calories without realizing it while they're putting dinner together, for instance.

It's also a way for you to stay on top of the big changes that are happening to you. First of all, good nutrition is paramount after weight-loss surgery; you'll feel the difference not just in how fast you lose but in your energy level. A quick look at your food journal will tell you whether you're really giving your body the very best fuels—lean protein, low-fat dairy products, and plenty of vegetables and fruits, or whether you need to renew your commitment to the program.

And let's say your weight loss slows down or stalls out, even though it feels like you're not doing anything differently. The answer will be in the pages of your food journal, making it very easy for you to correct. (These plateaus happen to almost everybody, by the way; for tips on pushing through, see page 258.)

Your food journal is also a good way for you to start to build a correlation between what you eat and *how you feel*. I encourage patients to review their food journals once a week; there's a lot of information in there! Wednesday you were a little short on protein—maybe that's why you felt so sluggish and low in energy at that late meeting. Tuesday you felt hungry all the time—and look, you were eating more refined carbs than you've typically been allowing yourself; maybe that's a sign that those foods don't satisfy you as well or as completely as some of the other choices available.

You'll also chronicle what your emotional state is when you find yourself gravitating toward food. Chances are good that you use food as medicine to "treat" something you're feeling. What this exercise will help you to do is to isolate those emotions so you can really address *them*, instead of simply masking them with food.

A notebook is good because it's portable, but it's easier than it's ever been to track foods online, with a program like FitDay.com or MyFoodDiary.com. These types of programs will count calories and give you a nutritional breakdown as well. (This is a good way to make sure your protein stays between 60 and 80 grams a day.)

Exercise. For the first six weeks, you won't be doing anything strenuous—and that includes serious exercise. But I do want my patients to walk twenty to thirty minutes every day, starting right when they get home, and to gradually increase the distance. It's usually better to take a couple of walks (one with the dog in the morning, one at lunchtime, and another in the early evening, for instance) instead of one long one that wears you out completely. By the time you arrive at your six-week postsurgical visit, you should be walking fairly briskly and covering some ground.

If you have joint problems, see Chapter 14 and talk to your surgeon about other kinds of exercise. Water exercises, for instance, are kind to sore knees and hips, and they're safe to do three weeks after surgery.

Check in with your support group. It's a good idea for you to reach out and take advantage of some of the support options available to you—from your friends and family at home and from the weight-loss surgery community.

Don't be surprised if you're ambushed by a lot of feelings in these early days. It's very normal to feel overwhelmed by this new undertaking or frightened that you won't be successful. You know intellectually that it's too early to see a difference in the mirror—but you feel so different, how can that change not be apparent to everyone around you? And if you've traditionally used food to medicate your depression or anxiety, you may find it hard to be without that crutch now, however unhealthy it may have been.

Surrounding yourself with supportive people is essential; talking to people who've been through the same thing can really help as well. People who had the same procedure are also a very good source of information about your new stomach and lifestyle—what is that terrible gurgling noise, anyhow? (See the box on page 133 for the answer.) Your surgeon's office should have at least one support group that you can attend.

A number of my patients have become part of an online community as well. Online forums are great for a number of reasons: They're available all the time, the people involved tend to be very supportive, and since so many people participate, they can be a tremendous source of knowledge and support. Of course, the advice you find here shouldn't be considered a replacement for bona-fide medical advice, and it's wise to take everything you read—including the occasional nasty comment—with a grain of salt. But in general they are a terrific resource.

Support from the WLS Community

Online Groups. Yahoo has a wide variety of support groups for WLS patients. Search OSSG (Obesity Surgery Support Group), and you'll find hundreds of subgroups on WLS and protein requirements, pregnancy, divorce, cross-addiction, the military, and about 240 other topics. **Obesity-Help.com** and **LapBandTalk.com** are both very, very active Web support groups, with thousands of active members. **LiteandHope.com**, for which Carnie Wilson is a spokesperson, also has active forums.

WLS Lifestyles Magazine. WLS Lifestyles is a print magazine covering all kinds of issues of interest to the WLS patient. (Their Web site, **WLSLifestyles.com**, has a very good searchable database of live support groups as well.)

Bariatric Radio. This online radio station, **bariatricradio.com**, archives its podcasts, so you can listen to shows on a variety of topics of interest to the bariatric patient, whether you're pre- or post-op.

WHAT'S THAT NOISE?

Many people report a lot of gurgling noises emanating from their stomachs after surgery.

It happens to both band and bypass patients, although for different reasons. The band makes it harder to burp, so once air gets into the stomach, the band acts as a valve, preventing its release. It is the passage of this air that creates the gurgles. Gas-X can help; avoid carbonated beverages, sipping with a straw, and chewing gum as well, which all contribute to swallowing air.

Air swallowing has a lot to do with the gurgling in bypass patients, too. But the real issue for them is that they're processing food differently now; specifically, carbohydrates are getting into the intestines faster and they're being digested differently—and this can create gas. It's harmless but uncomfortable, and it can be socially uncomfortable as well. See page 170 for some solutions.

Your New Pouch: An Owner's Manual

If you've had a gastric bypass, then what you'll really be doing in these early days is getting to know your new pouch. It doesn't require heavy-duty operating instructions, but there are a few things you should know to ensure that the two of you coexist peacefully. Here are some of them:

Dumping syndrome. Dumping syndrome—or what doctors call *rapid gastric emptying*—is a physical reaction to food that we often see in bypass patients.

There are two kinds of dumping syndrome: early dumping and late dumping. Early dumping syndrome takes place immediately after a meal; late dumping is more of a blood sugar reaction and happens a few hours afterward.

Early dumping syndrome: Ordinarily food—especially sugar—is digested over a period of time in the stomach. But if you've had a bypass, those sugars now move very quickly through the stomach and into the intestine, which responds by sending a large amount of fluid into the bowel. The resulting symptoms are, by all reports, unpleasant.

They may include:

- Rapid heart rate and palpitations

- Dizziness

- Sweating

- Nausea and vomiting

- Diarrhea

- Bloating

Foods that commonly make people dump are high-sugar foods (ice cream, cookies, cake, juice, candy, soda) and high-fat foods—especially those that combine fat with refined carbs, such as french fries, potato chips, and donuts. Milk and milk products make some people dump. So does too much fruit, although the fiber in fruit counterbalances the sugar for most people.

How you eat matters, too: Eating foods that are too hot or too cold and drinking liquids during your meals can cause problems in the beginning. But everyone is different and can tolerate different foods; the same thing that brings you to your knees might be very well tolerated by someone else. And it changes with time; you might be more sensitive in the weeks and months right after surgery.

You can see why surgeons sometimes list dumping syndrome as one of the "benefits" of bypass surgery. We don't want to see you sick—but high-sugar and high-fat foods are bad for your health and will arrest your weight loss. You have to listen to your body when it says "No, thank you!"

**The foods that make you dump
are the foods we want you to avoid!**

Even if you're scrupulous about avoiding these foods, something disagreeable may take you by surprise; most bypass patients do experience dumping syndrome once or twice. You'll know when it happens, although symptoms can range from the mild to the extreme. If you can, lie down and take deep breaths. Sipping water helps some people. But, in general, the only thing you can really do is ride it out—and in the future avoid whatever the food was that caused it.

Foods That Can Cause Dumping:

Ice cream	Sweet rolls, donuts
Pudding	Sports drinks high in sugar
Sweetened or fruit yogurt	Ice pops
Dried fruit	Cake
Candied fruit	Cookies
Frozen fruit or canned fruit in heavy syrup	Jelly or jam
Fruit juice	Soda, lemonade, or sweetened ice tea
Sugary cereals	Carbonated fruit drinks

Honey	Sherbet or sorbet
Table sugar	Maple syrup
Candy	Soup (taken without food)
Chocolate	Milkshakes
Chewing gum (not sugar-free)	Chocolate milk
Molasses	Bread-and-butter pickles, sweet
Syrups	pickles, and relish

Late Dumping: WLS patients also talk about late dumping, which essentially is a form of hypoglycemia: You take in sugar, and because the intestine is very efficient at absorbing sugar, the body miscalculates and releases a lot of insulin to cope, and so your blood sugar gets precipitously low. This can make you feel dizzy, weak, and really, really tired. It can also make you very hungry, because your body automatically will crave more sugar to counterbalance some of that excess insulin. So you can see why this is a cycle that can also lead to weight gain.

If this late dumping is something that happens to you often, pay careful attention to your food journal. You'll usually be able to spot the culprit—a few sips of juice with lunch, a piece of a high-glycemic fruit such as pineapple—a few hours before you began experiencing symptoms. Eating a lot of protein and limiting carb consumption to the complex carbs—whole grains and vegetables—is the best way to keep your blood sugar stable. Fruits are usually OK if combined with protein.

About 80 percent of people who've had a gastric bypass dump. The majority of them are happy for the help in avoiding the junk food. You might be looking at that list of foods and thinking that you could never live without something on that list. Interestingly, after the bypass those cravings really go away; most bypass patients will tell you that their tastes have just changed. Chocolate might cause dumping, but most patients just aren't interested in it anyway.

Band patients should take note: The list of foods that cause dumping is also a list of foods that will pass through a band easily and sabotage weight loss. And while band patients may not dump, they will get the fluxes in blood sugar that come from eating simple, high-glycemic carbs, and those fluxes will make you hungry. Hunger an hour or two after a meal is a sure sign that you had too much sugar with that meal. Check your food journal and adjust accordingly.

Don't smoke. Smoking after a bypass will cause an ulcer in your pouch. Notice that I didn't say that smoking "might" cause ulcers or "increase your risk" for ulcers.

If you smoke, you will get an ulcer. Period.

Don't do it—for your pouch's sake, if not for anything else. And while band patients don't face the same danger, I still highly recommend not smoking as part of your changeover to a healthy lifestyle.

Learn which meds are off-limits. One of my patients was admitted to the emergency room at 2 a.m. *on her wedding night.* Three years after her surgery, she'd forgotten the "no NSAID" rule, and had been popping Motrin for a couple of days to deal with her week-of-the-wedding stress headaches. The ulcer caught up with her on the first night of her honeymoon—a night she spent with me in emergency surgery, instead of in the Jacuzzi at a luxury hotel with her new husband.

Consider hers a cautionary tale—no matter how far out you are from surgery, certain drugs will always be unsafe.

Drugs that can damage your pouch include (check with your doctor before taking *anything*):

Advil	Bextra	Erythromycin
Aleve	Bufferin	Feldene
Amigesic	Butazolidin	Fiorinal
Anacin	Celebrex	Ibuprofen
Anaprox	Clinorinl	Indocin
Arthropan	Darvon compounds	Ketoprofen
Ascriptin	Disalcid	Lodine
Aspirin	Dolobid	Meclomen
Azolid	Equagesic	Midol

Motrin   Percodan   Tolecin
Nalfon   Ponstel   Uracel
Naprosyn   Prednisone   Vioxx
Orudis   Rexolate   Voltaren
Oruval   Tandearil
Pamprin-IB   Tetracycline

If you have questions about whether a medication is safe, call your doctor's office! It just takes a minute to ask—and it can save you some very real grief.

Band and sleeve patients don't have to worry as much about *which* meds they can take—but band patients do have other concerns, namely size. Large pills—even ordinary-size ones—can get stuck. I like it when my patients bring their meds with them to the pre-op visit so I can actually see the size of the pill. In general, if there is a liquid formulation of a particular medication, I recommend it. If not, be sure that you are allowed to crush the med, and remember that extended-release medications cannot be crushed.

Your pharmacist may be very helpful in reviewing your meds and suggesting changes before surgery. We have a pharmacist on our team who meets with our patients, but if your surgeon does not, you can review your options with the pharmacist at your local drugstore.

Alcohol. Alcohol is not absolutely denied after surgery, but there are a few things to remember.

First of all, alcohol affects people differently after bypass because the active ingredient is metabolized much more efficiently into your system. So even a little bit of booze will make you much more intoxicated than it would have before surgery, and it will take longer to clear. This is a bad situation. First of all, alcohol famously lowers your inhibitions—and not just the ones telling you not to dance on the table, but also the ones telling you not to order dessert.

Being a cheap date might not bother you that much, but bear in mind: This ultraefficient process also exponentially increases your exposure to the health risks of alcohol, including liver disease. And your new light-weight status also puts you at increased risk for accidents (vehicular and otherwise); you might have been able to drive home after a glass of wine at dinner before surgery, and now you won't.

Don't forget, alcohol is calorically expensive, too—and traditional cocktail mixers like tonic and cola are an absolute nightmare. Those excess calories can add up to weight gain, but they can also add up to poor nutrition. If you're eating a very-low-calorie diet, which is what you'll be doing after surgery, every calorie you take in matters. So I'm not happy to see the 150 calories in that beer nudge out a real food, i.e., something with actual nutrients in it.

Avoiding alcohol during your first year post-op makes sense from a psychological perspective as well. One of the things we're always watching out for is someone "trading" their addictions. If you previously numbed your feelings with food, it's important for you to have those feelings now, and to deal with them, instead of letting another numbing agent take food's unhealthy place.

THINGS TO DO DURING YOUR RECOVERY:

Follow your surgeon's post-op diet plan.

Sip lots of water—aim for 64 ounces over the course of the day.

Start a food journal.

Exercise daily.

Get 60 to 70 grams of protein a day.

Take your vitamins and supplements as prescribed by your doctor.

Go to your follow-up appointments.

Get to know your new stomach.

Check in with your support group.

||||||||||||||||||||||||||||||||||||||||||||||||||||||||||||||||||||||||||

CHAPTER ELEVEN

The Beginning of the Rest of Your Life

The Basics

"'There are children in Africa who'd be happy to have that dinner,' my mom used to tell us if we left anything on our plates. It took me forty years—and a gastric bypass—to realize that my obesity wasn't doing a darn thing for those kids. I send a check now; it works out better for everyone."

In the next chapter we'll get specific about what foods you'll be eating after surgery and when you can start adding them back into your diet. But before we go there, I want to go through what I call the basics. The basics are the central rules you'll be following as soon as you begin to recover in the days after surgery, and they will continue to be the dietary cornerstones of your postsurgical life, no matter which procedure you had. Because they're so important, I'm going to go through them in some detail. I don't just want you blindly following orders; in my experience compliance is much better when patients understand why they're doing what they're doing.

A good understanding of these basics should give you a sense of security as well. Not only will these be your guidelines in these early months, but the basics will always be there for you to return to whenever you feel shaky about your program.

Here they are:

- I will eat three small meals a day, made up of high-quality healthy foods, and one scheduled healthy snack.

- I will eat my protein first.

- I will not graze or snack between meals.

- I will drink 64 ounces of fluid a day.

- I will not drink with my meals or an hour afterward.

- I will exercise every day.

- I will take my supplements as prescribed.

- I will return for scheduled follow-ups with my doctor.

- I will get support when I am feeling challenged.

That's it. That's really all you need to know in order to get the best possible results from your surgery. I strongly suggest you photocopy the previous page and put copies wherever you'll see it: on the refrigerator, on your office bulletin board, in your wallet.

**If you stick with these basics,
you will be successful.**

It really is that simple. But there's quite a lot of information in that short list, so let's break it down together.

I will eat three small meals a day, made up of high-quality healthy foods, and one scheduled healthy snack.

This basic hits two important aspects of your diet after surgery: quantity and quality.

Let's talk quantity first. You're going to have to learn to stop eating before you feel full. Fullness may have given you a feeling of comfort before, but if you overeat after surgery, you'll probably feel quite ill, and you may even vomit. Over the long term, of course, you'll want to keep your portions small. Consume too much food and your pouch will stretch (band included); consume too many calories and eventually you'll begin putting on weight.

Portion control is the true goal of this surgery;
it is the only way to lose weight.

I strongly suggest weighing and measuring foods as a way to keep portion sizes under control. Right after surgery your stomach will only tolerate about an ounce of food. That's not very much—about the size of the tip of your thumb. The amount you can eat will increase, but your portions still will be much, much smaller than what you were used to eating before surgery. Ultimately you'll want to stop when you've eaten about a cup of food at every meal, or about 4 ounces.

The handiest measuring device available to you is your hand. Once you are eating normal foods, here's what a meal looks like: a palm's worth of protein and a palm's worth of complex carbs. In other words, a piece of chicken that could fit comfortably inside your hand and a small handful of green beans. This should be filling; if you have a band and are still hungry after a meal like this, you may need a fill.

A food journal will also keep you accountable. It bears repeating that studies show that people underestimate the number of calories they eat by between 50 and 100 percent. In other words, if you think you've eaten 800 calories so far today, the reality may be closer to 1200—or 1600! So keep yourself honest and measure out what you're going to eat.

And after you're done measuring, put the food away. Studies have also shown that when we're given large portions, we tend to eat more. One such study was done in healthy, normal-weight young men. When presented with bigger portions, the participants ate quite a bit more than they did when presented with smaller ones, which tells me that even people who don't traditionally have trouble stopping when they're full will eat more when they're given more.

So, as I mentioned earlier, trick your mind by using baby plates and baby forks and by cutting food up into baby-size pieces. Many of my patients choose to eat their meals from smaller salad plates and to serve individual meals from the kitchen instead of from family-style platters at the center of the table. These are good ways to keep portion control under control.

Finally, eating smaller portions more frequently may be the best option. I am okay with four meals and sometimes even five, as long as they are *scheduled* and *small*. You should not be grazing all day long, and you should not be overeating at any of these meals. The body is an efficient machine; it uses what it needs from a meal and stores the rest. Give it just what it needs and there won't be anything to store. Eating several small meals also helps avoid fluxes in blood sugar that make you ravenously hungry—a good thing, because it's when we're very hungry that we tend to eat the wrong foods.

ZEN AND THE ART OF MINDFUL EATING

I believe in mindful eating, which means chewing each bite carefully, savoring the aroma, the appearance, and the taste—as opposed to scarfing it down while watching TV. Doing this will make you feel full faster, and it will help you recognize when you get there.

But I also recommend that my patients take a single silent moment of contemplation before their meals to say a kind of grace. I personally take that moment to try to picture the people responsible for getting the food to my table. Was it grown on a beautiful farm, harvested, and sent to your local market—or was it created by a chemist at a big plant that spews ugly gas into the air? Was it food prepared with love, by your spouse, or at a local healthy restaurant—or was it the afterthought of an irritated teenager, sweating his way through his summer vacation in the back of a fast-food joint?

I don't want to feed my body with mystery meat that's been sitting for hours at an oily fry station. I want to picture nourishing food coming from a tranquil, organic farm, and I want to imagine that all the vitamins and minerals in that food are going to make my body healthy and strong. It might sound corny, but this visualization makes me feel like I am actually consuming all the love, care, and concern that went into getting that food to my plate—something you can't do with junk food.

Quantity is important, but *what* you're eating is just as important. I put a great deal of emphasis on what I call high-quality foods. What does that mean? It means foods that have not been processed, preserved, or otherwise messed with. Quality food doesn't come from a package or a box; it comes from the ground, or from a farm, or from the ocean. It doesn't have seventy-two ingredients you can't pronounce but one or two or three that even a preschooler could identify. Think chicken, eggs, broccoli—not partially hydrogenated palm oil and butylated hydroxytoluene.

Ideally the foods you'll be eating in this new phase of your life will be *whole foods*: fruits, vegetables, low-fat dairy products, lean sources of protein such as chicken, turkey, and fish, and whole grains. I think you'll be pleasantly surprised how much better you feel when you stick to these foods. You'll also be better nourished. When I first started practicing bariatric medicine, I was astonished to discover how many of my patients came in preoperatively with severe vitamin and mineral deficiencies. "How could they be malnourished, even on 4000 calories a day?" I wondered.

But when I looked at the food journals my patients provided, I understood. They weren't getting what they really needed from the food they were eating, and their bodies knew it. You can't trick your body: 1000 calories of junk isn't equal to 1000 calories of high-quality food. People deficient in iron have been known to eat clay and dirt; given how nutrient-poor the majority of the foods in the standard American diet are, it's no wonder that so many people are driven to eat and eat and eat. Their bodies are starved—not literally, but of what they need to keep healthy and strong.

Much of our hunger is driven by nutrient deficiency.

My general recommendation to my patients is that they buy the best food they can afford. I limit my family's exposure to pesticides by buying organic fruits and vegetables, and I choose hormone- and antibiotic-free meat. The phrases "free-range," "free-grazing," and "grass-fed" or "pasture-fed" are all indications that the animal was raised in a natural environment. These choices are a little more expensive, but I think they're worth it; there's no better investment in your health than to spend money on what you eat.

Bear in mind that how foods are prepared also affects how healthful they are. Grilling, poaching, broiling, and baking are all lower-fat preparation methods. Substitute whole milk with skim when baking, and oil with chicken or vegetable broth; replace some or all of the oil in recipes with applesauce or yogurt when you're baking. Add spices and lemon juice instead of olive oil or butter to flavor foods. Tricks like these can save you hundreds of calories over the course of a day, and chances are very good that you won't notice the difference. Even if your palate does give you a little resistance, commit to a change for a week; you'll most likely get used to it.

I love this way of thinking about food, because it means that people don't have to give up the things they truly love; they just have to tweak their diets a little to make them healthier. Make your omelet from egg whites and lower-fat cheese and add some vegetables instead of bacon. Make that taco with a whole-wheat tortilla or a low-carb multigrain wrap, and stuff it with ground turkey instead of beef. Top it off with fat-free refried beans, salsa, and low-fat yogurt, and you've got a much healthier, cleaner version than the one you used to eat.

"HELP! I CAN'T COOK!"

Preparing your own food as often as possible is the best way to make sure you achieve maximum weight loss. But some of my patients tell me that they don't know how to cook—or that they don't know how to prepare healthy, whole foods, although they had no problems frying something up for dinner before surgery.

If you genuinely don't know how to boil water, it's probably worth taking an entry-level cooking class at a community college near you. It doesn't need to be fancy, but I think you'll find that even simple foods benefit from being well prepared, and the basics are all things you'll be able to pick up in a few well-spent hours.

But the best way to learn to cook—or to learn to cook healthfully—is just to do it. There are thousands of WLS recipes on the Internet and a number of good cookbooks on the market aimed specifically at the WLS patient.

Some of the books my patients like include:

Recipes for Life After Weight-Loss Surgery by Margaret M. Furtado and Lynette Schultz

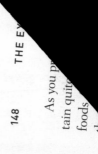

Eating Well After Weight Loss Surgery by
Bontempo-Saray

Before and After: Living and Eating Well After
Maria Leach

I also really like the *Eating for Life Cookbook* by
for WLS patients, though, so adjust portion sizes

I recommend buying one or two of these cookbooks, even if you're an experienced cook. You'll be preparing more of your own food than ever before, and boredom is the enemy of the WLS patient; even if you don't use the recipes, you can leaf through the pages and pick up some fresh ideas.

"No, I mean I *really* can't cook!"

In Houston and in many cities around the country, you can find services that will make and prepare healthy food and deliver it to you. Two days a week I go to work early and leave late, meaning that I eat all three meals at the hospital. On those days I have three healthy, hearty meals delivered to me by a company called Diet Gourmet. The service costs about $20 a day—and I think it's a great deal.

I will eat my protein first

After surgery you should aim for 60 to 80 grams of protein a day. That's quite a bit of protein, which is why we suggest that you eat your protein first; it's going to take a lot less to fill you up than it did before surgery, and when you're ready to stop eating, it will be crucial that you've gotten the protein you need.

And you do need it. Protein is the body's most fundamental building block; it's needed to make and fix every cell in the body. Your body needs a constant supply—and if it doesn't get it, your body will start to break down its own source of protein: muscle. That will make you feel nauseated and weak and leave you vulnerable to infection.

Good sources of protein include animal protein (poultry, meat, shellfish and fish, eggs), soy protein (edamame, tofu, miso), dairy products (milk, yogurt, cottage cheese, cheese), legumes (beans, chickpeas, and peanuts), and nuts. (See the Appendix on page 279 for a more complete list of protein-rich foods.)

obably can see from the list above, protein-rich foods often con-
a bit of fat. When possible, choose low-fat versions of high-protein
(such as skim milk, low-fat or non-fat cheeses, and lean meats); if
it's not possible, eat small portions (just a few nuts, for example).

It can be difficult to get enough protein right after surgery because your
pouch is still so small, so I usually recommend that my patients use supplements to get their full complement. You have a few options to choose
from. Soy protein powder is a good choice, but some people don't like the
taste; egg protein is another alternative, as is whey protein, which comes
from milk. Look for a supplement that gives you at least 20 grams of protein per serving, and beware of added sugars.

Once you're back to eating a wide variety of solid foods, I highly recommend that you get your protein that way, as opposed to relying on supplementation or bars or shakes. Don't get me wrong: A protein shake or bar is
a good fallback on a hectic day when you've fallen short—and we *all* have
those days—but I prefer that patients satisfy their nutritional requirements
by eating whole foods. Protein shakes in particular are a bad combination:
Not only are they high in calories, but they're liquid, so they pass through
the band or the pouch too quickly to keep you full.

Just because you're focused on protein doesn't mean that it's all you're
eating. In fact, the diet I recommend to my patients looks very much like
the Zone diet: In its simplest form, that means equal portions of low-fat
protein and good carbs, at every meal. The book *Enter the Zone* by Barry
Sears has a lot of good information about structuring a balanced diet.

Bad carbs are simple carb, the ones you find in sugar and sugar-filled
foods—the white or beige foods, as I like to call them. We call them bad
because they do bad things to your blood sugar. Candy, cake, ice cream,
potatoes, white rice, corn, peas, and white bread are high-glycemic, which
means that they spike your blood sugar quickly.

Low-glycemic foods—the good carbs—such as vegetables, whole-grain
bread, brown rice, and apples, cause a more gentle rise and fall in your
blood sugar, with none of the mood swings or ravenous hunger and cravings associated with their simpler counterparts. (I prefer glycemic load to
glycemic index, because it takes into account how rapidly the sugar hits
the bloodstream. Many good foods—watermelon, for instance—have a
high glycemic index because they have a high sugar content. But fiber

content slows the absorption of the sugar, which is how we arrive at glycemic load.)

As far as I'm concerned, keeping your blood sugar stable is the single
most effective way to free yourself from cravings and out-of-control hunger. That means sticking to good, low-glycemic-load carbs, eating them in
small quantities, and never eating them without protein.

Keeping your blood sugar stable should be
a priority.

Most good carbs are high in fiber, which is another bonus. Fiber helps
you to feel full, and, because it is not digested, it also helps to regulate your
bowels and has been shown to lower bad cholesterol. Fresh fruits and vegetables, beans, and whole grains are high-fiber foods.

So you'll eat good carbs in small portions, in combination with
high-protein foods—for instance, a piece of salmon on top of a green salad;
chicken breast and green beans; or yogurt (which has both protein and
carbs in it) with a few nuts on top.

I will not graze or snack between meals

America is a snack culture. We eat not just three square meals, but *all
the time.*

This is one of the reasons we struggle to control our weight. Snacking
tends to be mindless eating; it's something we do in front of the television
or in our cars. It also tends to be unplanned, which often means that we're
paying less attention to the quality or quantity of what's going into our
mouths than we should.

This behavior is especially dangerous for weight-loss patients. The benefit of your new stomach, whether you've chosen a band or a bypass, is that
you feel full after just a little food. But eating throughout the day instead
of at four distinct meals is a very effective way to sabotage this mechanism. If you feed your tiny stomach steadily, a little bit all day long, you're
going to stop losing—and eventually you'll start gaining. "It's just 100 calories," you might say to yourself—but when you've hit the refrigerator six
times between lunch and dinner, those calories really add up.

Band patients, please note: Walking around and then coming back to eat more of your meal when the food has passed through is not a meal; it's grazing. Eating should take twenty to thirty minutes. It shouldn't take less, and it shouldn't take too much longer.

If you find that you're very hungry between meals, then schedule a snack or a minimeal, and plan what you're going to eat in advance. That way you can spread out your calorie intake so that you're eating five 300-calorie meals instead of three 500-calorie meals (on a 1500-calorie-a-day diet).

Choose a protein-rich food, put it on a plate, sit down, and enjoy it. Please remember: When you're eating, you're *eating*—not standing up, not munching while you talk on the phone or flip through a magazine or watch television. And when you're done, you're done—until your next meal.

As I mentioned earlier, a food journal is another very effective tool to make sure you're only eating what you mean to eat: Those thoughtless snacks will seem much less appealing if you have to write each one of them down. Reviewing your food journal can also give you important information on which foods left you hungry for a snack an hour later; maybe cottage cheese isn't satisfying enough for your lunch without something else to accompany it.

I will drink 64 ounces of water a day

Our bodies are mostly made of water, and being well hydrated is essential to the body's proper function. The problem, especially in the early days after surgery when the pouch or the banded area is still swollen, is that it's hard to get enough liquids. You have to be vigilant and sip a little bit, every few minutes, all day long. Don't use a straw; straws force you to sip in a little bit of air with each pull, which promotes gas—more of something you don't need after WLS.

"I don't like water!" some of my patients tell me. I can't really relate to this: I think a cold glass of water is one of the most refreshing things in the world. But if you don't, you still can keep your fluid intake up with a few tricks.

- Some people prefer to take their liquids at room temperature; if you're one of them, leave your beverages out of the fridge.

- Make a giant pitcher of unsweetened, caffeine-free herbal tea and allow it to chill overnight.

- If your stomach can tolerate citrus, add a squeeze of lemon, lime, or orange to your water glass. (One of my patients drops a frozen strawberry into the bottom of her glass in the morning and then refills the glass over the course of the day.)

- Crystal Lite, diet Kool-Aid, and sugar-free iced-tea mix are other alternatives that you can mix in to flavor your water.

I will not drink with my meals or an hour afterward

Drinking with meals often makes people dump, but that's not the only reason it's a bad idea. You should forgive the metaphor, but drinking with your meals after surgery is sort of like flushing a toilet. Liquid will help the food to leave the pouch very quickly—taking your full feeling with it.

Imagine pouring the contents of your lunch into the drain of a sink; it's going to go down much more slowly if you don't chase it with water, right? In order to extend the amount of time you feel full, refrain from drinking for about fifteen minutes before a meal and for about an hour and a half afterward. This applies equally to the band, the bypass, the DS, and the sleeve.

I do, however, recommend "water loading"—drinking a cup of cool water about fifteen minutes before eating. This curbs appetite and can help you to eat less during the meal.

I will exercise every day

Exercise is enormously important after bariatric surgery. It's your best weapon against dangerous blood clots immediately after the procedure and an A-1 metabolism booster after that. You see, not only do you burn calories when you're exercising, but you burn more calories than you ordinarily would after exercising, too. And exercise helps to build muscle, which burns more calories—even at rest!—than fat does.

But that's not all it does; in fact, scientists often refer to exercise as the wonder drug. Among other benefits, exercise can fight depression, improve mood, lower bad cholesterol, increase good cholesterol, improve insulin control, enhance self-esteem, and even give you a better sex life! Most important, it is scientifically proven to help you live longer. The Framingham Heart Study, a well-known research project that followed the residents of a town for more than forty years, showed that an exercise program extended lifespan by almost four years.

Bariatric patients have some specialized exercise issues, but *everyone*, no matter how big, can find a form of exercise that works for them. There's no physical issue you can't work around with a little creativity and some dedication. The studies have clearly shown that weight-loss surgery patients who work out for thirty minutes, five days a week, lose significantly more weight than those who do not exercise.

You'll find lots of advice for dealing with exercise issues in Chapter 14.

I will take my supplements as prescribed

This basic is especially important if you've had a malabsorptive (or partially malabsorptive) procedure such as the bypass or a DS switch. The areas in your GI tract where certain crucial minerals ordinarily would be absorbed have been bypassed; unless you supplement your diet with these minerals, you run the risk of deficiencies.

This is serious business: Many of these deficiencies can not only make you feel sick and weak, but they can cause permanent and irreversible damage. Calcium deficiency can lead to osteoporosis; iron deficiency can give rise to fatigue, hair loss, and anemia; zinc deficiency can lead to brittle nails and hair loss; vitamin A deficiency can lead to night blindness; vitamin D deficiency can lead to calcium deficiency and osteoporosis; vitamin E deficiency can lead to poor wound healing; vitamin K deficiency can lead to easy bruising; vitamin B_1 deficiency can lead to neurologic disorders; and vitamin B_{12} deficiency can lead to fatigue, anemia, and neurologic disorders. And those are just the highlights.

So it is absolutely crucial to comply with the supplementation program prescribed by your surgeon. The supplements you're taking will likely include:

Calcium. Calcium is essential for bone health: Without a steady supply of enough calcium, your bones will develop small holes. Eventually this weakening of the bones leads to osteoporosis, which dramatically increases your risk of bone breakage from even a minor fall. This in turn can lead to major surgery and even permanent disability. Unfortunately, bypass surgery and DS dramatically reduce your ability to absorb calcium, so you'll need to supplement every day.

It's important to note that all calcium supplements are not created equal—especially for bypass patients. Calcium carbonate needs stomach acid to be absorbed; since you'll have less stomach acid after your bypass, calcium citrate is a better choice for a WLS patient.

I recommend the bariatric calcium citrate chews from Bariatric Advantage because it is hard to find a chewable calcium citrate in most stores, but the brand is up to you: Just make sure *calcium citrate* is the active ingredient.

I know I said that I'd prefer for my patients to get their protein from food sources, but please don't make the mistake of thinking you can eat your calcium. Foods such as cheese, tofu, and broccoli *are* good sources of this important mineral, and I hope you'll eat them. But it would take *four pounds* of broccoli to deliver 1200 milligrams of calcium. Even if eating that much broccoli appealed to you, weight-loss surgery patients simply can't eat that much food. In this case, there's no substitute for a pill.

Vitamin B$_{12}$. Neither is there a substitute for a B$_{12}$ supplement. B$_{12}$ is poorly absorbed in bypass patients. Deficiencies can cause symptoms such as anemia, fatigue, and a tingling or numbness in the hands.

Vitamin B$_{12}$ cannot be taken in pill form; it needs to be absorbed rather than swallowed. All my bypass and sleeve patients take sublingual B$_{12}$ in the form of drops that you put under your tongue every day. (Shots are also available, but they're less convenient and they need to be administered monthly.)

Iron. Iron is a vital mineral that can be poorly absorbed after a bypass, resulting in fatigue and anemia and even some hair loss.

But too much iron can be bad for you, too, causing constipation and even heart disease. Some surgeons check iron levels and supplement as needed, but I recommend that everybody take iron for the first three months. After that, I recommend that only menstruating females continue, but I do check iron levels at follow-up visits.

If you do have an iron deficiency, I recommend taking iron and combining it with vitamin C for better absorption. Do not take iron with your other supplements—*especially* your calcium—because the two may bind and thereby affect absorption.

Ferrous sulfate is the most common store-bought iron, but it can be very constipating. I suggest using ferrous gluconate instead. (There are a number of good companies out there making vitamins and supplements for bariatric patients. The ones we use in our practice are made by Bariatric Advantage. You can find them at BariatricAdvantage.com.)

Multivitamin. It's pretty rare to get perfect nutrition in a day—taking a multivitamin makes sure that your bases are covered. And *everyone* should take one. Although bypass and DS patients are at special risk, we see a lot of vitamin and mineral deficiencies in patients *pre-op*. That tells me that the general public probably could do with some supplementation, so I tell my band and sleeve patients to take their vitamins, too.

I used to tell my patients that they could take any chewable multivitamin, but I began to see certain B vitamin deficiencies in my patients that these multivitamins didn't address. Prenatal vitamins were my original choice, but the formulations vary widely, and I couldn't guarantee that my patients were getting thiamine and the B vitamins. I now recommend that they switch to products formulated specifically for weight-loss surgery patients such as the ones made by Bariatric Advantage.

It's still a good idea to keep a bottle of the chewables, such as children's Flintstones, in the house, though, in case there's a gap between when you run out and the arrival of your reorder; I'd rather have you take something second-best than not take anything at all.

Choosing a supplement. When purchasing supplements, look for the initials USP (testing organization U.S. Pharmacopoeia) or words such as "release assured" or "proven release," meaning the supplements are easily dissolved in a short period of time.

Don't forget to take them! In general, the easiest way to remember to take your vitamins is to leave them out in a prominent place; the kitchen counter, for instance, or on a tray on the breakfast table. In a house with children, though, all supplements should be kept out of sight, in child-safe bottles on a high shelf.

Take your supplements at the same time every day, before or after you do something you always do, like brushing your teeth in the morning or washing your face at night before bed. One of my patients keeps a full set of supplements in her office; that way if she forgets to take her supplements in the hectic bustle of getting her family out the door in the morning, she has another chance when she gets to her desk.

Don't self-prescribe! Having this surgery means that you're going to need to take more than the amount recommended for the general population. Follow your surgeon's instructions. And don't add any medications or herbal supplements without informing your PCP or your surgeon; you want to avoid adverse drug combinations or those that might interfere with the absorption of your supplements.

I will return for scheduled follow-ups with my doctor

It's essential to maintain a relationship with your surgeon's office, even after you've settled into your new life. If you have the band, you'll need to return to your surgeon for adjustments to your fill; if you had a bypass, you'll need annual blood testing to make sure you're not experiencing any deficiencies.

But don't be shy about touching base between appointments! Call if you're not sure about a new medication or over-the-counter drug. Don't ignore abdominal pain down the line, either; a postsurgical complication can arise at any time.

It's especially important to go back to your doctor when things aren't going well. I know it's emotionally hard to do so—in fact, a bariatric patient I know called it "slinking back, tail between [his] legs." But it's essential—and crucial to do it at the first sign of trouble. I ask my patients to do a big reevaluation of their diet and exercise program after five pounds gained and to call the office after ten.

One patient came in to see me after she'd gained back quite a bit of weight, more than half of what she'd lost to get to her goal weight. As gently as I could, I asked her why she'd waited so long. "I didn't want you to feel like you'd failed," she told me. I was touched that her first worry was for me—but trust me, your doctor is not going to feel like a failure if you come back when you're struggling. We want to be able to give you everything you need to succeed, and that includes the support you need when the going gets tough. (We made an appointment for the patient with Mary Jo Rapini, our therapist, and another with our dietician, and encouraged her to come back to the support groups. With a little help, she did indeed get back on track.)

There's something else to think about: You may be used to calling your family doc for run-of-the-mill gastroenteritis, the routine bellyaches that can happen to anyone. But after weight-loss surgery, your GI tract has changed in ways that only your bariatric surgeon will understand, so your first call should be to your surgeon's office.

**Any severe or nagging pain after WLS may be
something related to the surgery.**

Things can go wrong, even years down the line. For instance, after the bypass or DS, a bowel obstruction from a twist can happen years later; symptoms include bloating, cramping, and vomiting. Your primary care doctor may not know how to handle this, but your bariatric surgeon will get you in quickly and fix it immediately, and time is of the essence.

Pain and burning in your upper/mid-belly could be an ulcer or the result of gallstones, which are common after extreme weight loss. If you develop mid- to right-upper abdominal pain and nausea, call your surgeon.

And if you have a band, call your surgeon for an appointment ASAP if you have vomiting and reflux—especially if pain is severe. It may be as simple as just pulling out some fluid, but it also may be a sign of a slip, and surgery might be necessary.

I will get support when I am feeling challenged

First of all, you don't just need support when you're feeling challenged—you need (and should have) support all the time.

You can find that support in any number of places, whether from a family who agrees to keep cookies and chips out of the cupboards, from friends who shop for new clothes and trade healthy recipes with you—even from a dog who loves that morning run as much as you do and waits by the door with her leash.

But having a good support system is especially important when times get tough. I guarantee it: There will be moments when you feel overwhelmed by the challenges ahead of you. If you find yourself thinking, "I can't do this," pay attention, because what you're really saying is "I can't do this *alone*."

The good news is that you don't have to. It might take a little work to figure out what you need—and then how to get it—but with a little initiative, you can make it happen. For instance, this came from one of my patients: "I stopped losing, about ten pounds away from my goal weight. When I saw that I'd gained a pound or two, I told my husband I wanted my birthday present early and splurged on two sessions with a personal trainer. He motivated me and taught me some tricks, and the scale started moving again."

Reach out and get yourself the help you need, whether that's someone to talk to, someone to work out with, or someone to take care of your kids for an hour. Some sources of support include:

Support groups. Go to the support groups provided by your surgeon's office—even if you feel like you don't need to. These support groups are usually led by a medical professional—a dietician, nutritionist, bariatric nurse, or mental health counselor. They're a place to trade information and get some encouragement from people who—unlike your friends and family—know *exactly* what you're going through.

If your surgeon doesn't hold support groups, or if they're not convenient for you, try to find another bariatric surgery support group in your area. You can call another surgeon's office and see if you'd be allowed to join one of theirs; you can also search for support groups in your area on Web sites such as ObesityHelp.com. Some bariatric patients start their own groups. Support groups can be wonderful, with one caveat: If the group isn't moderated by a medical professional, I'd advise you to be very cautious about the medical advice you hear there.

Joining a group like Overeaters Anonymous or WeightWatchers may also be helpful because they tend to have more frequent meetings (OA even holds meetings by telephone and online), although you may get more benefit from groups that work specifically with bariatric patients. Many bariatric support groups publish a telephone list so that you can reach out to other members of the group in a time of difficulty. If yours doesn't, consider asking someone in your group to be your buddy—someone who will offer inspiration and encouragement by phone or over tea when you're having a hard time in between meetings.

It's never too late to go back to a support group! Many of the faces in our monthly group are a few years out from surgery; in fact, the further away you get from your surgery, the more you may benefit from a refresher course in the basics and the camaraderie of those who have walked a mile in your shoes. And don't forget that your needs may change as your life changes. "I stopped going to support groups about eighteen months out; it felt like it was the same stuff, over and over again. But then my mom died, and I could see that I wasn't in a good place, so I made myself go. I didn't talk too much; just being with people who'd had surgery helped me to remember that gaining weight wasn't going to bring her back," one of my patients confessed. Take your emotional temperature frequently, and reach out for that extra help when you need it.

WHAT TO LOOK FOR IN A SUPPORT GROUP

One of my patients told me that the friends she's made in the WLS community are so important to her that she considers them to be a collateral benefit of the surgery, almost as important as the weight she's lost. By all accounts, it is a wonderful experience to be in the company of people who really understand what it means to be a weight-loss patient.

But not everyone has such a positive experience, so it's important to choose your support group wisely. In general, the bigger the group is, the less time each individual member will get. Some people prefer the comparative anonymity of a big group, but if you want more specific attention, a smaller group will be a better fit.

Specialized support groups are also a good idea. Our practice has a support group that specializes in nutrition education and another one that's focused on exercise. We've found that the issues people deal with immediately after surgery are different from the ones they have down the road, so we've got a special group set up for people who are six months out or more. We also have a very small support group for people who are more than a year out; in order to join that group, you have to commit to attend every single meeting for six months.

When I hear about "bad" support group experiences, it's usually because the discussions often got stuck in a very negative mode. There's certainly no rule against complaining; of course, talking about complications and stumbles is an important part of the experience. But there should also be some focus on education, on goal setting, and on moving forward. That's really the moderator's job; if the group is unmoderated or if the moderator isn't effective at moving the discussion toward the positive, it might be time for *you* to move on.

Online communities. Visit the message boards on sites such as ObesityHelp.com, and you'll see tons of posts like this one: "Having a hard day—made some bad choices last night and I'm feeling pretty bad about myself."

Keep reading, and you'll find a flood of posts in response, filled with sympathy, good wishes, and encouragement. You'll also find tons of stuff of interest to people who've had WLS—the best-tasting protein powder, stories about dumping syndrome, before and after pictures, clothing swaps.

The benefit of these online communities is that they're enormous and operate pretty much around the clock. Some of my patients have gotten very involved and are constant presences on these sites; others are too shy to post but benefit just from reading what others have written.

I've said it before, but it bears repeating: Be careful. Unless someone's a nurse or a doctor, they've got no business dispensing medical advice, and you've got no business taking it. And, unfortunately, some people take advantage of the anonymity of the Internet to be unpleasant; don't engage in arguments that seem more personal than productive.

Friends and family. The bariatric community isn't the only place you can find support. Simply taking the time for a manicure or a walk with a friend can completely refresh your outlook.

And if you're having a hard time, say so! If you're the caretaker, or "the strong one" in most of your relationships—and many obese people find themselves in that role—it can be hard to ask for help. You may also be finding yourself leaning more heavily on people than you're used to as a result of the surgery, and you may feel hesitant to ask for more. But you'll take better care of others if you have what you need to take care of yourself, and I think you'll be pleasantly surprised by what happens when you get up the courage to ask.

Be as specific as you can about what you need. "Would it be possible for you to take the car in to the shop tomorrow so that I can exercise after work?" Note that this request is phrased in the form of a question. Ask—and listen to the answer! If the answer is no, don't get discouraged; see if there's something else that will work.

Get creative! See if a neighbor will do a child-care trade with you so that you can have a little alone time with your partner. If you're tired of your own cooking and find yourself joining in when everyone else is ordering in, ask a coworker to bring an extra healthy lunch with her tomorrow and promise to return the favor on Thursday. (Unless she's also a bariatric patient, you'll need to adjust portion size accordingly.) If you're feeling trapped and exhausted, switch chore lists with your spouse so that you burn some calories cleaning the garage while he makes dinner and gets the kids ready for bed.

In other words, support can come from lots of places—even from some unexpected ones. Don't hesitate to reach out and to get what you need. You have taken a tremendous step toward better health, a step that enriches everyone around you, and you deserve to be reinforced and encouraged for making it.

||||||||||||

Those are my basics, but you may want to add your own personal rules to that list. Remember: It is often easier to say "never again" than to allow yourself to cheat, and this is where you may decide to add a personal basic to the list. I'll give you an example that one of my patients shared with me. The small executive cafeteria at the place where she works is filled with foods that aren't good for her, such as fried chicken and fish sticks and gooey macaroni and cheese. After her bypass, she made a vow to herself that she would bring her own lunch from home, and for a long time—the length of time it took her to lose more than 120 pounds, to be exact—she did.

But after she'd reached her goal weight, she got a little lax and started nibbling around the edges of the buffet table: a bite or two of mac and cheese, a drumstick with (most of) the batter scraped off. For a while it was okay—and then she started gaining weight.

She came to see me, and we talked about the ten pounds she'd put on. "What's changed about your eating habits?" I asked her, and she knew the answer right away. So now she has gone back to one of *her* personal basics: "I don't eat from the cafeteria; I eat what I've brought from home." Not surprisingly, those pounds have come off again.

So give this some careful thought: Maybe you need to swear off fast-food joints or certain trigger foods—forever. Maybe you'd benefit from a reminder not to eat in front of the television or while you read. If those are your personal basics, they should be added to the list.

Remember, the basics are always here for you. Photocopy the list on page 142 and post it anywhere you need it. Write the basics down on Post-its and plant them around the house. Amend them, with your own goals and achievements.

And what if you make a not-so-good choice? Get right back up again, dust yourself off, and make a better choice the next time—not tomorrow, but at your very next meal.

CHAPTER TWELVE

Your Diet Schedule After Surgery

You probably won't be very hungry in the week immediately after surgery. But eventually your appetite (reduced though it may be) will return. What you'll find in this chapter is a schedule of what foods you can introduce back into your diet, and when it's appropriate to do so. This schedule is designed with two purposes in mind: to allow your new stomach to heal without strain, and to get you used to the new foods—and amounts—you'll be eating in the weeks and months to come. To keep it simple, I advance my bypass, band, and DS patients on pretty much the same progression.

You may notice that what you read in these pages deviates from what your own bariatric program recommends. This is what we have found to work best for our patients, but I strongly suggest that you stay with your surgeon's recommendations.

Week One

Most patients report very little hunger in these early days. At the hospital you'll be given broth, juice, and water. You'll continue with those when you get home, limiting the juice to one cup a day. If you had a bypass, dilute the juice well to prevent dumping (many bypass patients can't tolerate juice at all at the beginning).

Once home, I recommend that you start to incorporate some protein in the form of shakes and powders, but the consistency of the liquids you're eating still should be very loose, like water. (If it fits through a straw, it's okay.) You can dilute protein shakes with skim milk or add protein powder to clear broths. Try strained miso soup, a good source of protein in its own right. (Miso paste is available in many supermarkets and at Asian specialty markets. And miso soup is incredibly easy to prepare—you just swirl a tablespoonful into a cup or two of water, heat, and drink.)

Because you're eating so little, I'd advise you to eat often: 2 to 4 ounces of liquids—sipped, not gulped—every hour that you're awake. You'll reduce the frequency when you move to more solid foods.

Weeks Two and Three

Break out the blender! After one to two weeks, you can move on to puréed foods with a slightly thicker texture (think of baby food). To prepare, add water or a little skim milk to the food as you blend it until it reaches the desired consistency.

Strained cream soups and yogurt-based shakes and smoothies are good choices. A little cream of wheat with protein powder added or grits thinned with skim milk—even tuna and chicken salad that have been blended until there are no distinct pieces remaining—are also good options. Sugar-free pudding and gelatins are okay, too; add protein powder for added nutrition. Well-mashed scrambled eggs or egg substitute and puréed low-fat cottage cheese are also good protein sources. Some people can tolerate well-mashed bananas and applesauce.

Everything you eat at this stage should be completely puréed, with no chunks remaining. Even tiny solids, such as seeds, can give you trouble in these early days. If it can't fit through a fine-mesh strainer, don't try to eat it.

Again, you're not eating very much, so I recommend that you eat four or five meals a day, of about 2 to 3 ounces each. Don't be surprised by how little food it takes to fill you up! In these early days your stomach is still very small. It can only hold about 1 ounce of food, which means that just 2 or 3 teaspoons may be enough.

IS IT SOFT ENOUGH?

Could you eat it if you didn't have any teeth? If the answer is yes, it's probably soft enough.

Weeks Four Through Six

By your third to fourth week, you'll be ready to move on to what we call "mushy" and "crispy" foods. This may be sooner than what you've seen elsewhere; I prefer for my patients to move away from purées as soon as possible. Why? The bulkier the food, the more full it makes you feel; it's very easy to eat too many calories when everything you're eating is blended into oblivion. Once the healing process has begun, it's time for you to begin experimenting with mushy and crispy foods.

I recommend eating three meals a day, of about 4 ounces per meal, with one small (1/4-cup to 1/2-cup) high-protein snack. This is about what you'll be eating going forward, and for the rest of your life. Stop eating when you're full!

CHANGING TASTES

Don't be surprised if some of your favorite foods don't taste as good to you as they did before your operation. One of the weirdest side effects of bypass surgery is that foods actually taste different to some people afterward. (We don't see this with the band.)

Some patients report a coppery taste; others say that foods they used to love just no longer taste good to them. Sweet things, fruit in particular, seem to taste sweeter—often unpleasantly so.

Take advantage of this alteration in your taste buds to try new foods, even those you think you don't like. You may be pleasantly surprised by how they taste to you now!

Mushy foods. Mushy foods are what they sound like—very soft foods. Some examples include:

Eggs: scrambled, soft-boiled, or in the form of egg salad. (Fried egg yolks also are okay, although high in fat; you may have trouble with the rubbery white of a fried egg at this point.) Since eggs are high in fat, you'll want to explore substitutes like Egg Beaters and All Whites.

Dairy products: soft cheeses and cream cheese, low-fat yogurt, skim milk. (Avoid ice cream, whole milk, cream, full-fat cream cheese, and whipped cream.)

Legumes: beans, lentils, and peas, which are terrific sources of protein and fiber. You'll want to cook them really well and purée them into soups, refried beans, or whole beans that have been well mashed. Peanuts are also legumes, and peanut butter is a good source of protein, but it's high in fat, so use it sparingly (opt for smooth at this point).

Animal protein: tuna salad, chicken salad, ham salad—essentially any kind of meat that can be spread on a cracker. You'll want to purée (or chop very small) them for the first weeks, and avoid any kind of meat—including SPAM—that contains gristle, as it can get stuck in an unpleasant way. I suggest that you use low-fat or non-fat mayo to speed weight loss, and choose tuna packed in water as opposed to oil.

This is not scientific, but I have noticed that a lot of patients report difficulties with beef and pork, even when puréed, so add them back cautiously, and not earlier than the fifth week. I would rather patients avoid beef and pork anyway, and I recommend only lean cuts of these meats if they're well tolerated.

Meat in general can be troublesome: Choose moist and juicy meats— chicken thighs, for instance, as opposed to breasts. Grilling food takes out the moisture, making the food more difficult to swallow (sorry, George Foreman); rotisserie chicken goes down much better. No matter what method you use, *don't overcook.*

Fruits: By the second or third week, you may feel up to trying some peeled fruits, such as apples and pears. (Careful! Fruits are sweet and can cause dumping in some people.) By week four, you may be up to trying some citrus, such as grapefruits and oranges; eat just the meat, avoiding the connective membranes and the pith, which can get stuck.

TINY, TINY BITES

One of the hardest habit changes after surgery is learning to eat slowly, chewing and swallowing each small bite well before taking another.

But it's a habit you're going to have to acquire, because inhaling your food after weight-loss surgery will make you sick—fast. Food will get stuck at the opening of the stomach, and it will come back up. Eating too fast can also cause dumping syndrome after bypass.

Cut up each piece of food to the size of a pencil eraser. Don't load your fork. Chew your mouthful many times—until it is completely liquid in your mouth—before swallowing. Chewing thirty times per bite is the goal. This is especially important for more fibrous foods such as meat.

You'll also want to slow the rate at which you eat—two or three mouthfuls a minute, as opposed to five or six. It may help you to put your fork and knife down between bites.

Cut food into small pieces, take small bites, and chew well before swallowing.

If something gets stuck, try slowly sipping a glass of water with a teaspoon of meat tenderizer mixed into it.

If you find yourself vomiting frequently after you transition back to solid foods, something is wrong. You may have made the transition too soon; try returning to a liquid diet for a day or two.

Remember: Even one bite too many can lead to heartburn, nausea, and vomiting. You may be eating too fast or too much at one sitting—some foods will swell slightly in the pouch, which can lead to the problems above. Stop eating well before you feel full; if vomiting after meals is a persistent problem for you, stop eating after a single ounce and wait a few minutes before trying again. Fullness will feel different to you than it did before surgery; instead of a feeling of comfort, you'll have a sensation of pressure in the center of your chest and right below your rib cage.

As a reminder, don't drink with your meals. You also should not lie down immediately after you eat. If you've had a bypass, you should be avoiding foods that contain sugar or you may experience dumping syndrome. You won't be able to tolerate every food; if you always feel sick after eating a specific food, it's a sign that it doesn't agree with your new tummy.

If your vomiting continues, return to the liquid diet you were on in the first week. If you can't transition to solid food after that, you must call your surgeon.

Crispy foods. To know whether something can be categorized as crispy, all you have to do is ask yourself, "Would this disintegrate if I put it in water?" Melba toast, toast, crackers, baked tortilla chips, and pita chips—these are all examples of crispy foods. Whenever possible, choose the whole-wheat or multigrain version of these foods; otherwise you're just getting a lot of simple carbohydrates.

Foods to avoid. In this early stage you'll want to avoid anything too fibrous. Raw vegetables, such as carrots and celery, for instance, can get stuck and cause discomfort. Even cooked veggies such as green beans can give you trouble; if you must have them, cook them well past al dente, and take tiny, tiny bites.

Fried, salty snacks—think potato chips and Doritos—are completely out of the question. Forever, I'm afraid.

Adding foods back in. Everybody has foods that don't agree with them—foods that make them dump, foods that make them throw up, foods they can no longer tolerate the taste of, and foods that tend to get stuck.

Foods that give a lot of people problems include raw vegetables, rice, pasta, bread, carbonated beverages, and tough, stringy meats. But I've heard it all: One of my bypass patients lost 100 pounds with no intolerances, except for an immediate and violent reaction to *cilantro*, of all things. So you'll have to figure out what works—and doesn't work—for you.

Add foods back slowly—in other words, don't sit down to a meal of four or five "new" foods, or you'll never figure out which one is making you sick. Something that makes you sick now may be okay in a couple of months, though, so keep checking back.

And don't misunderstand the signals that your pouch is sending. If one or two bites of a food makes you feel uncomfortable, that doesn't necessarily mean that you can't tolerate that food; it might simply mean that a bite or two of it is sufficient to fill you up!

IT'S OKAY TO WASTE IT!

Never has the saying "Your eyes are bigger than your stomach" been truer than in the months after weight-loss surgery. That's going to mean that sometimes even the small portion on your plate is going to be too much for you to finish. If you were raised in the clean plate club, then it can be hard to tip the remainder of what's on your plate into the garbage, but it's something you're going to have to learn to do. Eating too much will not only slow your weight loss, but it will hurt!

Adventures in the Bathroom

"I haven't thought this much about toileting since my kids were little!"

Abdominal surgery means changes in your digestive tract, which might mean more excitement in the bathroom than you'd reckoned for. Some of the most common problems include:

Soft stools. You may have between one to three bowel movements a day. They'll be soft until you start eating more solid foods. You may also experience diarrhea: If you do, cut out cow's-milk products and foods high in sugar, if you're eating them (although you shouldn't be eating the latter!). Diarrhea shouldn't be persistent; if it is, contact your surgeon, and make sure you're drinking enough fluid to make up for what you're losing.

Frequent, soft stools are to be expected long-term with the DS but not with the band or the bypass.

Constipation. On the other end of the spectrum, you may find that the comparatively-low-fiber diet you eat in the early days after surgery means that you're going less frequently and that your stool is hard. Increase the amount of liquid you're drinking, and exercise—natural movement does help. You can try prune juice (not more than half a cup!), which acts as a natural laxative—but this may cause dumping in bypass patients. I would also add a fiber supplement such as Benefiber to your diet, but remember that it won't work unless you are drinking plenty of water.

If the problem persists and you're very uncomfortable, talk to your doctor about recommending a laxative or stool softener such as MiraLAX.

Flatulence. Everyone has gas in their digestive tract. If you've had a bypass, your digestive tract is much shorter than most people's. As a result, you may find that your gas both smells worse and is expelled more forcefully than it used to be.

If gas is a problem, first look at your diet. One common culprit contributing to gas in bariatric patients is lactose intolerance, or an inability to tolerate cow's-milk products. (Gastric bypass "unmasks" lactose intolerance—a condition that between 30 and 50 million Americans suffer from—but it does not cause it.) Give up milk products and see if the problem is alleviated. (You can replace dairy products with soy products—soy milk, soy yogurt, and soy cheese—or with products designed for people who are lactose intolerant, such as Lactaid.) Don't forget to read your labels! Some breads, dry cereals, and soups contain small amounts of lactose; look for whey, lactose, non-fat milk solids, buttermilk, malted milk, margarine, and sweet cream or sour cream in the ingredients list.

People with lactose intolerance usually can still eat products made from goat's milk (seriously: don't knock it until you've tried it). And unsweetened cow's-milk yogurt is pretty well tolerated, even in people who have trouble with lactose; the probiotic bacteria in it may also help with symptoms.

Sugar alcohols (sorbitol, mannitol), which are often found in dietetic products, can also cause gas; avoid them and see if you experience relief. Another culprit is swallowing air. Avoid chewing gum, hard candy, and carbonated beverages, and make sure that you're chewing small bites of food very well before swallowing, especially if you have a band.

If the problem continues, talk to your doctor. I suggest patients take probiotics, which are beneficial bacteria that can help to process food (my

favorite is Primal Defense by Garden for Life), and Beano, a digestive en-
zyme. Natural chlorophyll, available at health food stores, and simethicone
(such as Mylicon or Gas-X), available at the drugstore, can also help. If
these remedies don't work, you may want to consider a product called Dev-
rom, an over-the-counter internal deodorizer that neutralizes gas odor, so
at least your family won't kick you out.

Weeks Four Through Six

By four to five weeks after surgery, you'll be back to a "normal" diet,
which is to say that you should be able to eat pretty much everything your
family eats, if only in small portions, and without sugar.

Be patient, bypass patients: It may take months for you to tolerate ordinary foods. Band patients may have the opposite problem: Once the swelling goes down, you may not feel like you have any restriction, until your
first fill. It's important to make good choices now.

Hopefully everyone has used your surgery as an excuse to take a step
toward healthier eating. If you're not the head chef, though, and find yourself surrounded by junk, you're going to have to go your own way. You don't
have a lot of room in your new stomach—if you don't get good nutrition,
you're not going to feel good. And, even with the severely limited size of
your new pouch, it is still possible to consume enough high-calorie foods
that you can significantly slow your weight loss, and I know you didn't go
through all this not to lose.

You should be eating about 4 ounces at a meal (2 ounces of protein and
2 ounces of low-glycemic-load carbohydrate). I like my patients eventually
to end up at about 1200 calories a day. You're not eating as much, so make
every bite count!

IT'S OKAY TO ENJOY IT!

Many obese people find it uncomfortable to enjoy their food—they associate loving food with doing something bad such as breaking a diet or going off program. But just because you're losing weight doesn't mean that you need to feel deprived. There's no reason not to eat really, really great foods—you're just going to be eating them in much smaller portions than you ever ate them before. And, for the first time in your life, you're going to feel satisfied.

Grocery Shopping, the Bariatric Way

If there's nothing good to eat in your house, you'll wind up making bad choices. Planning ahead will be an essential part of your success in the months and years to come; smart grocery shopping will ensure that you have what you need on hand to make good choices. That's one reason we encourage you to stock your pantry with lots of nonperishable items. There are going to be days when you don't make it to the market, but you always should have enough healthy, satisfying foods in the pantry to put together a delicious low-calorie meal, even if you haven't been to the grocery store in a week.

Here are some good guidelines:

- The outside aisles of the store are the ones that contain the foods you'll want to fill your cart with: fruits and vegetables from the produce aisle, low-fat dairy from the dairy case, lean protein from the butcher's counter. Avoid the center aisles.

- Don't shop while you're hungry. It may be a cliché, but it's true; you're protected from a lot of those impulse buys if you've eaten a small meal or had a protein shake before you head out.

- Use the meal planner below to figure out what you're going to eat over the course of the week, and then make a list of everything you'll need to make that happen. (You can swap days within the week and freeze prepared meals if something comes up.)

- If you tend to get tempted by packaging and new products while you're shopping, promise yourself that you won't buy anything that's not on your list.

- If you don't want to eat it, don't buy it. It's much easier to say no to unhealthy snack foods in the supermarket aisle than it will be when you're looking through the cupboards later that night.

- Read behind the label. For instance, "unsweetened" doesn't mean there's no sugar in a product; it simply means that the manufacturer hasn't added any. Check: What's there already can be substantial.

- And pay attention to serving sizes. Just because it comes in what looks like a single-serving package doesn't mean it contains one serving; in fact, many "individual" packages actually contain two or more servings. Of course, your own serving sizes after surgery will be quite a bit smaller even than what's recommended.

- Stock up! It's sad but true: It costs a little bit more to eat healthfully. You can offset some of those costs by buying extra when a healthy food you like is on sale. (When you cook, make enough to freeze additional individual portions that you can defrost in a pinch.)

- Eat the colors of the rainbow (and you know I don't mean Froot Loops). Whenever possible, substitute a food with color for a white one—multigrain bread for white, a sweet potato for a white potato.

- If it comes from nature, it's okay; if there are twenty ingredients you can't pronounce on the side of the box, put it back. Processed food isn't just unhealthy; it will slide easily through your pouch and interfere with weight loss.

Meal Plan

Use this chart to figure out what you're going to eat over the course of a week, then make a grocery list of everything you'll need.

	Sunday	Monday	Tuesday	Wednesday	Thursday	Friday	Saturday
Breakfast							
Lunch							
DInner							
Snacks							

Grocery List

This isn't a comprehensive list, but it contains many of the staple foods you'll be eating.

For the freezer:

Skinless chicken breasts
Pork tenderloin
Lean ground beef
Sugar-free fruit or fudge pops
Frozen fruits and vegetables

For the pantry:

Vegetable, chicken, and beef broth
Low-sodium, low-fat soups
Canned tuna in water
Canned crabmeat or salmon
Balsamic vinegar and flavored vinegars: sherry, raspberry, tarragon, and
    so on
Light mayonnaise
Low-calorie, low-fat salad dressings
Canned tomatoes
Salsa
Canned beans (chickpeas, black beans, kidney beans)
Whole-grain pasta (quinoa, kamut, whole-wheat)
Carnation Instant Breakfast (no sugar added)
Protein powder
Whole-grain crackers (Wasa, Finn crispbreads, and so on)
Nuts (almonds, cashews, walnuts)
Seeds (pumpkin seeds, sunflower seeds)
No-sugar-added jam
Splenda or another artificial sweetener
Agave nectar (a low-glycemic sweetener available at health food stores)
Stevia, which is one of the best natural sweeteners
Crystal Light or sugar-free Kool-Aid

For the fridge:

Eggs

Egg substitute/egg whites

Skim or low-fat milk

Low-fat yogurt (I prefer the unflavored Greek type, which also has
more protein. If you prefer yours sweetened, consider adding a
spoonful of agave nectar or a no-sugar-added jam.)

Low-fat or non-fat cottage cheese

String cheese

Laughing Cow spreadable cheese wedges

Low-fat mini Babybel cheese rounds

Deli meats: turkey, lean ham, chicken

Tofu (the silken type is great for smoothies; firm tofu is better for cooking)

Fresh fruits and vegetables, including broccoli, spinach, carrots, cabbage, string beans, snow peas, cucumbers, tomatoes, avocadoes, salad
greens, peppers, squash, cauliflower, asparagus, onions and garlic,
bananas, oranges, mangos, cherries and other berries, apples, pears,
lemons and limes, cantaloupe, honeydew, watermelon, peaches, apri-
cots, grapes, and so on

A NOTE ABOUT TOFU

Tofu is easy to digest, a great source of protein, and very inexpensive compared
to meat. But many of my patients scoff when I suggest it; they have visions of
sandal-clad hippies eating it with a side of alfalfa sprouts. I think there's so
much resistance because people just don't know what to do with it. I hope a
little information can entice you to pick up a block and give it a try.

The most important thing to know about tofu is that it doesn't taste like
much. That's a drawback for a lot of people—until they realize that it can be
made to taste like a lot of things. Tofu will take on the flavor of whatever it's
served with, whether it's a spicy Thai coconut milk sauce, your uncle's famous
secret-recipe barbecue sauce (watch the sugar!), or raspberries and vanilla
extract in a silken pudding dessert. Use it in place of chicken or fish in your
favorite recipes, and try it as a high-protein dessert option.

Firm tofu is the easiest to cook with and has the most satisfying texture. You can make your tofu even firmer by wrapping it in a clean cloth and placing a heavy dinner plate with an additional weight on top of it for forty-five minutes. Pressing the liquid out of it this way will give it a chewy, more meatlike texture. Tempeh, also made from soybeans, is another satisfyingly chewy meat replacement.

Soy products have come a long way in the last few years, and there are lots of options. Look for soy hot dogs, soy granola, soy butter, soy cheese, and soy yogurt, as well as soy pasta and soy-flour pretzels at your health food store.

The change in the way you eat after surgery starts as you wheel the cart down those aisles. WLS shouldn't necessarily mean giving up all of your old favorites; in many cases you simply have to choose a lower-fat, lower-calorie version.

For instance:

- Use low-fat, or non-fat dairy options (milk, yogurt, cream cheese, cottage cheese, sour cream) instead of full-fat versions

- Use reduced-fat (part-skim) cheese instead of full-fat versions

- Try sorbet or low-fat or fat-free frozen yogurt instead of ice cream

- Replace cream-based pasta sauces (such as Alfredo) with tomato sauce or olive oil and vegetables

- Replace ground chuck in hamburgers and meatloaf with ground turkey or extra-lean beef; stretch the meat with finely chopped vegetables

- Replace white pasta with whole-grain alternatives (whole-wheat, quinoa, kamut)

- Replace white rice with brown rice, quinoa, millet, or unpearled barley

- Replace sugary cereals and granola with unsweetened whole-grain alternatives (shredded wheat, oatmeal, bran flakes)

- Use chicken and turkey on sandwiches; look for reduced-fat ham and lean roast beef

- Replace bacon with turkey bacon or Canadian ham

- Buy tuna packed in water, and use low-fat mayonnaise to prepare it

- Replace eggs with egg whites or an egg substitute, or use one whole egg and supplement with whites

- Avoid eating chicken or turkey skin

- Choose tenderloin (beef and pork) over other cuts; trim the fat before cooking

- Choose whole-grain or sprouted-grain English muffins and breads

- Try ginger snaps, fig bars, animal crackers, and vanilla wafers—they are better choices than other cookies; watch quantities and sugar!

- Favor baked or reduced-fat potato chips and light popcorn—they are better salty snacks than their full-fat counterparts; try soy nuts or a small quantity of almonds, walnuts, or peanuts instead

- Try reduced-fat or non-fat puddings, sugar-free fudge pops, and no-sugar-added juice pops, which can satisfy a sweet tooth

- Choose low-fat or reduced-fat salad dressings, or use a spritz of olive oil and lots of lemon juice instead

AVOIDING TRIGGER FOODS

As you begin to eat more and more foods, you may notice that some give you more trouble than others in terms of portion control. If you find that eating a particular food seems to stimulate your appetite or start you off on binge-type behavior, it may be a trigger food.

It can be hard to work around trigger foods. You can try to portion-control them (buy single servings or put appropriate portions into zip-top bags), but if that doesn't work, it's probably best to say good-bye to them altogether: Don't buy them, and don't allow them in the house. Find something else that you enjoy without having the uncontrollable urge to eat more of it.

A New Way of Thinking About Food

As you have seen over the course of this chapter, what you eat—and how much—are going to be radically different after your surgery. Enjoy these new foods and this new way of eating. The change may take a little getting used to, but you'll start seeing results pretty much immediately.

In the next chapter, we'll talk about another big piece of the puzzle: Changing the way you *think* about food.

CHAPTER THIRTEEN

The Honeymoon Period

"It feels like the best dream I've ever had. I go for hours without thinking about food, for the first time in my life!"

"I felt really scared and depressed after surgery; I missed food and the way I used to eat."

"My only regret is that I waited so long to have surgery. I wish I could have my thirties back; this time I'd go through them as a thin person!"

In the first six to eight weeks after surgery, you'll be getting back to normal. But a lot will have changed about "normal." You'll be learning to eat in a completely unfamiliar way, and you'll be incorporating exercise, plenty of water, and vitamins into your daily routine. You may be able to come off of some of the medications you've been taking to control your diabetes, hypertension, and other diseases associated with obesity. And you will be losing weight! More, perhaps, than you've seen come off in a lifetime of dieting, and certainly much faster.

The six to nine months after bypass and DS surgery are what's referred to as the honeymoon period. (We'll discuss what's going on for band patients during this time on the next page.) This period of time is usually characterized by extremely rapid and significant weight loss—and by a sense of euphoria. (Typically we see about twenty pounds come off the first month, and then ten pounds each month after that.)

What you thought was completely impossible is now happening. You'll start to get the double takes and comments like, "Wow, you look terrific!" There's a high probability that you will hit the century mark—100 pounds lost—during this time, depending on your starting weight and co-morbidities. And you'll probably begin to *feel* much better—less creaky in the joints, more energetic, and sexier than you have felt in years. It's a heady time, and you should enjoy every minute of it.

This is not to say that you won't have to put effort in; you will. The people who are *most* successful long-term are the ones who use this honeymoon period as a chance to press the "do-over" button on a lifetime of unhealthy food choices and habits. They're the ones who equate having surgery to winning the lottery and who realize that they must spend every penny wisely; the ones who realize that surgery gives them a tool to change their relationship with food and their behaviors and attitudes toward it. The long-term successes are the people who use the procedure to put an end to being "victims" of obesity and take the opportunity to own up to every bite they put in their mouth.

The honeymoon period is limited—something that you should realize going into it. It does not last forever—even though many people treat it as if it does and then wonder why they never achieved their goal weight. If you understand that this is just a window of opportunity, you can maximize your weight loss during this period, putting you on the path toward long-term success.

This is not true for the band patients. In fact, these first few months may leave band patients wondering whether any surgery was done at all. The band requires adjustments every month, and the true calming of your hunger does not occur until the band is adequately filled. So we typically see only three to five pounds of weight loss a month. In other words, band patients learn early what the bypass patients come to know after the honeymoon is over: You still have to work at weight loss.

In this chapter, we'll talk about what to expect during these months—and how you can use this time to make sure you're losing for a lifetime.

The Not-So-Romantic Side of Rapid Weight Loss

The weight is coming off, and that's a great thing, but some of the things that come along with rapid weight loss can be less, uh, glamorous. Not every individual experiences these side effects—but it's good to know in advance that there is a possibility.

Gallbladder problems. Problems with the gallbladder are common with any serious weight loss, no matter how that weight loss is achieved. Individuals suffering from obesity have a high rate of gallstone formation anyway, and many of my patients already have had their gallbladders removed. (If your gallbladder already has been removed, gallstones won't be a concern for you after surgery.)

Some bariatric surgeons remove the gallbladder at the same time they perform weight-loss surgery. I prefer not to put my patients through any surgery that's not strictly medically necessary; instead I generally put my patients on a medication called Actigall, which helps to prevent gallstones, for six months after surgery. (Because weight loss is much slower in band patients, I don't require this of them.)

Many people with gallstones do not have symptoms, but common signs and symptoms of a gallbladder attack can include nausea, vomiting, and mild or severe pain in the pit of your stomach or the upper right quadrant of your belly, which may even radiate to your right upper back. Many people report feeling chest pain similar to that caused by a heart attack. At the first sign of these symptoms, you should call your doctor right away. You may require surgery to remove your gallbladder.

Hair loss. Most people experience hair loss with rapid weight loss, however they lose it. Hair loss usually occurs in the first four to eight months after surgery, during the time of greatest weight loss.

This can be an upsetting side effect, and you may swear you have enough hair on your bathroom floor to create a small dog, but I have never seen a single bald spot. In other words, the hair loss may be noticeable to you but not to others.

This too shall pass: The hair will stop falling out eventually, and it will grow back. In the meantime, there isn't much you can do. Nutrition is your best weapon, especially protein and vitamins. Some patients report that Nioxin shampoo is helpful, as are biotin tablets or powder; I have also heard that flax seed oil helps. Make sure you are getting your vitamins and minerals, as zinc and iron deficiency can cause hair loss.

I also recommend that you put as little stress on your hair during this time as possible; avoid perms and dyes and heavy styling. You may also choose to go with a shorter haircut during this time to take some weight off the hair and to give it the appearance of greater body on top.

Skin changes. Sometimes patients report that the texture and appearance of their skin is different than it was before the weight started coming off. Some develop acne or dry skin for the first time in their lives.

The best thing you can do for your skin is to keep your nutrition as excellent as possible, always making sure you're getting at least 70 grams of protein a day, and faithfully taking your vitamins. Over-the-counter remedies including moisturizers and acne preparations may help; you may need to change your skin-care regime to accommodate your "new" skin. A trip to the dermatologist may be in order if your symptoms are extreme.

If you're feeling overwhelmed by these prospects, know that my patients are unanimous in their agreement that the weight loss is worth whatever side effects they encounter. Stay on track and keep your nutrition solid; there's a healthier you to strive for and achieve.

Band fills. If you've opted for a band, you'll spend the early months after surgery getting your band fill exactly right. It's more of an art than a science—and sometimes it can be a frustrating process for the patient. Stick with it through the fine-tuning, and you'll reap the rewards.

When you come in for a fill, your doctor will ask you how much you are eating, if you are having reflux, and if you are vomiting. Your answers will determine how much fluid is added or removed. During a fill we numb the area with an anesthetic and then inject saline solution into the port. It doesn't take very long, and patients report it to be relatively painless. (Some surgeons will do the fill under an X-ray while you drink a dye solution to determine the size of the opening.)

Most surgeons like to fill the band slowly and frequently. I, for instance, like to see my patients every month for six months. (As I mentioned above, we're looking for about a three to five pound loss a month.) This allows the patient to learn to eat more slowly and to chew more. Once the patient gets used to a certain level of restriction, we can go tighter.

People often think that they'll lose more weight with a tighter band, but the opposite is often true. In fact, research done by bariatric surgeons in Australia indicates that patients do much better if the bands are not too tight. The reason for this is simple: If the band is too tight, then good foods—lean proteins, such as chicken and fish, and high-fiber, low-calorie foods, such as fresh fruits and vegetables—can't get through. What can? Chips, cookies, chocolate shakes—all the foods you must avoid in order to lose weight and gain a healthier life.

**You should feel *some* restriction,
but you should also be able to eat healthy foods.**

The goal is to get you to what we call the green zone. In the green zone you get full easily with about 2 to 4 ounces of food, and you stay full for a good while, so that every meal isn't a battle with your willpower. There should be little to no vomiting (unless you eat too fast or don't chew properly), and you shouldn't have reflux or chest tightness.

I suggest to my patients that they turn to their measuring cups and scales to determine whether their fill is appropriate. The rule of thumb: You should feel satisfied—not full to the point of pain or illness, and not ravenously hungry, but perfectly content—after a 4-ounce meal.

Band fills can be tricky. A perfect fill suddenly can feel too tight for no apparent reason—my patients tell me that even barometric pressure can affect how it feels, which is great if you want to predict the weather but not if you want to live normally. Your band may feel tight in the morning and loose at night. Sometimes the band doesn't feel tight right after the fill but kicks in a few days later. Sometimes it feels tight in the office but fine when you leave. (You see what I mean about it being an art form?) One common explanation for a sudden feeling of tightness is eating too fast; even if a stuck piece of food eventually gets through, it can cause a little swelling and inflammation.

But once we find your sweet spot, you should continue to enjoy weight loss of one to two pounds a week, as long as you are following the Basics.

If your weight loss stalls or you feel like you are able to eat too much, your band can be readjusted. Most patients undergo three or four fills the first year, but once it's right, you should be able to enjoy being "fill-free" for quite some time; some people will even go a year. The fluid in the band can evaporate out over time, though, so a yearly fill is not a bad idea.

If you're not feeling full, or if you only feel full for a short time after getting a fill, your band might be leaking. If we can't withdraw the same amount of fluid we put in, there's a leak. If there is any question, we can also check by injecting dye into the port and using an X-ray to see if any leaks out.

If your band fill allows you to eat 4 ounces at a sitting but you're still not losing weight, you have to ask yourself some tough questions: What am I eating? Am I eating a balanced diet with an emphasis on lean protein and small portions of complex carbohydrates? Have some of the foods I ate before surgery snuck back into my diet? Am I drinking with my meals and pushing food through so that I end up overeating? Am I snacking during the day? Is all of my eating mindful eating, or am I grazing throughout the day? Am I consuming enough water or opting for high-calorie beverages like that mocha frappuccino? Am I exercising at least thirty minutes daily? Am I getting at least eight hours of sleep every night? Am I taking my vitamins daily?

Keeping a food journal remains the best way to monitor yourself honestly. (As I mentioned before, FitDay.com is a great online journal.) I would also suggest that you take your journal results to your dietician, who can help you figure out how many calories you actually need over the course of the day—and then help you to create a diet plan that ensures you're taking in fewer than you burn.

Stay on Track!

No matter which surgery you choose to have, remember: This is your time to lose. Eventually your body is going to catch up, and your metabolism will slow down. So, even though it's possible to sneak in some extra calories and still see those numbers on the scale decrease, *don't do it*. Slowing yourself down now really jeopardizes your chances of reaching your goal weight. Take advantage of your lack of hunger and the quick weight loss you're experiencing to get as close as you can to your ideal weight. Use this period to establish good new eating and exercise habits.

TURN OFF THE TV

At the risk of sounding like I'm micromanaging: Turn off the TV.

There is a direct correlation between how much television a person watches and their weight, and it's not surprising. The television is the source of *a lot* of negative messaging about food. In fact, I recently was shocked to see a commercial for Snickers during an episode of *Big Medicine*! If you're moving toward healthier eating habits, you don't need to hear about a new fast-food burger with six strips of bacon on it! It's time for us to control our own minds.

Plus, watching TV while you are eating is an old eating pattern—a mindless one—and you have to start making new eating habits now in order to be successful. Remember, mindful eating is what we're after. Every bite counts!

What's Driving You to Eat?

This losing period also gives you an opportunity to look at the way you have always thought about food—and what about that mind-set needs to change, if you're to achieve your new, healthier life.

We've talked about obesity and genetics, and we've talked about the prevalence of the inexpensive, high-calorie, high-fat, low-fiber foods that trigger the genetic propensity to this disease. But there is also a strong psychological component driving obesity, and coming face-to-face with your relationship with food is really the only way to ensure that you achieve the success you deserve. I worry greatly about the patient who tells me he has no idea how he became obese. In order to win over this disease, you will have to get some insight into how your eating habits failed you in the past.

As I've said over and over, the surgery is only a tool. It is not a magic bullet designed to save you from yourself. If you use food in any way other than fuel, or if being significantly overweight feels "safer" to you than having a normal BMI, then you will find a way to get around any weight-loss surgery—I guarantee it. Restriction and malabsorption are no match for your mind.

> **If you do what you've always done,**
> **you'll get what you've always gotten—**
> *even after surgery.*

I hesitated before leaping into this topic; people suffering from obesity feel judged already, and I know that most of my patients have done twenty times more soul searching than the general population. But at the same time, I know that asking and answering the tough questions presented in this chapter—doing what we call "the head work and the heart work"—has helped a lot of people to put self-destructive, sabotaging behaviors behind them.

> **The more you know about the factors that**
> **contributed to your disease, the more successful**
> **you'll be after surgery.**

You had surgery on your stomach, not your brain. And, as they say in the WLS world, that was the easy part.

Before I jump into the heart of this chapter, I have to stop and thank a colleague of mine, Jamie Carr, RN, whose work in the bariatric community is unsurpassed. I am fortunate to have her on my team, and my patients are fortunate to have her in their corner. In addition to being a phenomenal bariatric nurse, Jamie specializes in aftercare support with an emphasis on behavior modification. Much of what you will read in this chapter is the result of the years of work she has done with literally thousands of weight-loss surgery patients, and which she has been willing to share with me.

Ending Emotional Eating

Identifying emotional eating patterns actually is pretty simple. Food is fuel. Anytime you're eating to satisfy an emotional need instead of a physical one, you're eating inappropriately.

We call this "head hunger." Head hunger is what you're suffering from when you've more than satisfied your stomach—but still find yourself heading back to the fridge or to the cupboard because you aren't satisfied. You may feel tired, stressed, angry, depressed, or lonesome, and because food has always been your friend, you yearn to reconnect with it. Breaking this pattern of emotional eating is going to be essential to your success. But it can be very difficult, and it requires a real level of commitment and a lot of hard work.

The first step is for you to identify the emotion (or emotions) that is pushing you toward food. Literally—as you open the refrigerator door—you have to stop and ask yourself, "Is my belly hungry? Do I need fuel? If I don't need fuel, then what is it that I am I feeding? What am I feeling right now?" The simplest way to do this is to leave a small journal or notebook by the fridge, snack drawer, or cupboard that used to hold the foods you reached out for before surgery.

Note in your journal if you're tired, stressed, anxious, or feeling lonely or depressed. Make mention of any precipitating events—an upsetting phone call, a cancelled plan, something sad on television, a disappointment—whatever it is that is causing you emotional angst. You might feel surprised at how trivial the trigger seems, but if you feel it's connected, make a note of it.

Then at least you know what you're dealing with. In truth, dealing with those emotions is the only real road out of your pain. After all, you can throw food at your upsetting feelings all day long, but food will never make them go away. If you'll permit the medical metaphor: It's the wrong medicine. Food won't make you less lonely or less angry. It *can't*—it's just food. All it can do is mask those feelings or numb them and distract you in a very temporary way.

Of course, used this way, food will also make you overweight and sick. Meanwhile, you're not getting the help you really need, so that your underlying emotional needs remain unfulfilled. That's just going to lead to more emotional eating, and, ultimately, to more weight gain.

Stop. Identify. Choose.
In the long run, emotional eating just makes
you feel worse.

This is where the head work comes in. In truth, this is hard to do by yourself, which is why we so strongly encourage weight-loss surgery patients to ask for help. Talking to someone about those underlying feelings is a very good way to resolve them. Get in touch with the counselor your surgeon works with or share your feelings with the people in your support group. You'll soon see that many people are experiencing the same feelings and frustrations as you and that there is a great deal of comfort to be found in knowing you are not alone. Talking with someone who is qualified to help can make all the difference in the world.

To guide you in this head work, I recommend working through the following questionnaire. These are just some of the questions put out to members of our support groups in the past, with the intention of helping them connect their eating patterns to their feelings. (It's never too early to begin this work, by the way; you don't need to have had the surgery to start looking more closely at your relationship with food.)

Emotional Eating Questionnaire

Answer as honestly as you can—this is for you alone. Take as much time and space to answer as you need:

What are your first memories of food?

How was food used in your home? Was it a bribe? Did your parents withhold food, or certain types of food, as punishment?

What are your first memories of your body?

Do you remember being teased in your family because of your weight? Were you ever yelled at or made to feel shame because of it?

Was one of your parents obese? If so, how did the rest of the family cope with that?

While you were growing up, was anyone in your family coping with an addiction—to food or to something else (drugs, alcohol, shopping, sex, gambling)?

Who over the course of your life has had the most influence on the way you relate to food, your body, and your weight? List the people who had the most positive influence and those who had the most negative influence.

What is your most painful memory about food?

What foods do you miss since your surgery?

Can you name some of your food-related fears?

What do you struggle with when you make food choices? When do you struggle the most?

What emotion is most likely to cause you to eat? Which other emotions do you try to seek comfort from or cover up with food?

When is this most likely to happen? What time of day or after what precipitating event?

What are the things about yourself that you are most proud of or like best about yourself?

What are the things about yourself that you are most ashamed of or like the least?

Can you imagine yourself at a healthy weight? Do you know what that would look like or how that would feel? What do you think stands in the way of making that happen?

Does anything about the idea of yourself at a healthy weight frighten you? If so, what? Be honest.

Is there anything you can think of that would help you to create a more positive environment for yourself? What obstacles are in the way of making that happen?

Do you feel that you take good care of yourself, physically and emotionally? If not, why not? What's missing?

What—other than food—has made you feel better about something that's hurt or upset you?

Line Up Your Weapons

Without a deeper understanding of why you're eating emotionally, the behavior will never stop. But some behavioral fixes can also help you to make sure you don't sabotage your weight-loss efforts. If you've watched *Big Medicine*, you may know that Mary Jo Rapini uses an analogy in her practice and in our support groups: "You're a hunter, and the urge to eat inappropriately is something you have to hunt down and kill. What are your weapons?"

I love this image. First of all, it reverses the way we usually think about coping with food cravings or the urge to eat emotionally. Instead of seeing yourself as subjected to the whims of something larger than yourself, something completely out of your control, the image of a hunter puts the control in *your* hands: You're lying in wait, ready to stalk and destroy anything that threatens your progress. These weapons, of course, are best developed in peacetime—when you're not actively craving food—so that in a crisis they're there when you need them.

And the more weapons you have, the better. Some days it's going to feel like you're stuck in the bunker, outnumbered by cravings. You're going to have to shoot more arrows than you even thought you had in your quiver. As Mary Jo says, "That's because they're still messing with you. They don't know yet that you're going to demand to be taken seriously. That's why you need a show of force."

So what's in your arsenal? Here are some of the strategies we've heard from patients in our practice that we highly recommend:

Call someone. Twelve-step programs encourage everyone to have a sponsor, someone a little further down the road who will answer the phone and talk you through a rough patch. This is a great idea for everyone—and it doesn't even have to be an official sponsor. Making connections at live support group meetings is a great resource for finding people that "get it"; sometimes just talking things through is all you need to avoid that bag of chips.

Exercise. Pretty much every weight-loss book tells you to take a walk when you feel a craving coming on. In truth, it works—because exercise triggers the same pleasure chemicals that eating does. Try to replace the urge to eat inappropriately with physical activity; it will help you to discharge the emotion that was driving you *and* help to make you more fit, and that's a cross-addiction I can support!

Meditate. I never cease to be amazed by the power of the subconscious. Thinking evokes a very real response in your body. For instance, when you think about something bad that happened to you, your body will release stress hormones, as if you were reliving that experience. And for too many of us, thinking about painful things drives us—often without realizing it—to what we perceive as the comfort and safety of food.

We have to learn to control our minds, and meditation is one very effective tool to help us do so. It's been used and written about for thousands of years, but it's only recently that Western medicine has begun to embrace its amazing effects. There are now hundreds of well-respected scientific studies from venerable institutions such as Harvard University showing the benefits of meditation for treating all kinds of diseases.

You can buy one of the thousands of instructional books and tapes on the market, but the fundamental principle actually is very simple: Meditation is learning to clear your mind. It's like teaching a dog to stay. You tell your mind to stay and give it something to focus on—your breath, a word, or a mantra. Like a puppy, it will get distracted and try to run away; the art of learning how to meditate is guiding it gently back until it begins to obey.

The principle is a simple one, but it is one of the hardest things in the world to achieve. You sit, you clear your mind, you concentrate on your breath. Suddenly you think, "Hey, look at this. I'm doing it! I'm meditating. No problem. This isn't so bad. It's easy. Easy like Sunday morning. Wait, who wrote that song? Was that Lionel Richie? I think so. And he did that 'Endless Love' song, right?" And then suddenly you're not meditating anymore—you're wondering what happened to the girl you went to that movie with so many years ago.

But just because it's difficult doesn't mean you won't get it. I suggest doing the following meditation technique at least once a day—ideally, twice—once in the morning, and again at night.

Sit comfortably. You don't need to be contorted into a yoga pose; if your mind is constantly thinking about the pain in your knees, true meditation will be impossible. (On the other hand, you don't want to be so comfortable that you fall asleep.) I suggest sitting in a chair with your back straight.

Take several deep, slow, and deliberate breaths. Feel the air enter your nostrils and fill your lungs from the bottom up, as if you were pouring water from one pitcher into another. Once you start to feel at ease, imagine that there is a cloud of bright white light floating above your head and beaming rays straight into the crown of your head. With each breath, draw the light into your body, and follow it as it flows through you. Feel its relaxing and healing energy in the muscles of your face. As it flows down your neck and back, feel the muscles there loosen and relax. Feel the light flow into your chest, filling your heart with peace, and follow it as it travels down your arms, through your abdomen, and down your legs. Once it has gone through your body, imagine that this beautiful white light is surrounding you in a protective cocoon.

Safe in this protective ball of light, begin to meditate. Choose your focus point—a flame you stare at softly, a word like *peace*, or just a sound, like the time-tested "Om." You don't have to say it; just think it. Or simply follow your breath as it goes into your nose, down your windpipe, into your lungs, and out again.

For fifteen minutes, try to concentrate on your focus point. Do your best, but don't be hard on yourself. If your mind wanders, simply return it back to your point of focus; eventually it will calm down and come under your control.

If you do this daily, you will start to feel an inner peace I cannot explain, and you will also notice that you are developing real inner control. The more you do it, the more you will be able to take this peace and control into your daily life.

Use an affirmation. Many cultures have a version of this practice, which is essentially the repetition of a simple saying over and over. It's been done for thousands of years because it works!

Pick something powerful to say to yourself, and then repeat it as often as you can. Repeat it as you prepare breakfast, as you shower, as you drive to work in the morning, while you're exercising, and as the last thing you do before you go to bed at night—anytime you have a minute, and certainly anytime you feel shaky or in need of some support. Post it as a reminder at home and at work.

Your affirmation should be something positive, something that makes you feel powerful and successful, such as "I am beautiful," "I am healthy," or "I am lean." (Of course, it can be anything that works for you.) It should be in the present tense. As you repeat your affirmation, you'll probably notice that the meaning changes for you.

If you're a visual person, a photograph may be a more effective affirmation. One man I know pasted his own head on a picture he cut out of a magazine so that he looked at his head on top of the body he was working toward every morning when he shaved.

In support groups we often ask the group to offer their favorite affirmations, and then we vote on which one the whole group will use for the month to come. It can be very powerful at the end of the month to hear what feelings a particular affirmation or mantra brought up for people. Propose something similar for your support group (or online support group).

If you're a person of faith, you may decide to use your prayer time as affirmation and to ask God for help when you need it. Make the choice that works for you and gives you the most comfort.

SPEAK THE TRUTH

"One's not going to hurt."

"I deserve a reward."

"I'm so stressed; a cookie will help."

Your messages may be different, but you'll recognize the little voice of sabotage in the statements above. In support groups we suggest that people come up with statements of truth that contradict and correct these messages, such as "One *does* hurt," or "I deserve to be healthy and to achieve my goal weight," or "I'm stressed; going for a walk will help."

Write down some of the things you say to yourself when you're in self-sabotage mode—and some of the truer things you can say, next time, in response.

Write in a journal. As far as distractions go, writing in a journal is one of the very best ones, especially if you can address some of the emotional issues that are driving your craving to eat.

Be honest in your journal, and dig down deep. This is how you will begin to identify patterns of eating and how they correspond to events, emotions, and/or emotional triggers in your life. In addition, being able to have a "safe place" where your feelings are not judged is very important. Many individuals who have lived with obesity tell me that they never felt heard or understood; using a journal is one way you can begin to have a voice and to strengthen the core of who you are.

Love yourself. I find that many people who suffer from obesity (and from the stigma attached to it) aren't very good at loving themselves. Here are some little ways you can love yourself:

Give yourself a pedicure. Blog. Turn on a favorite song and dance your heart out. Clean something. Fix something. Organize a closet. Catch up on your scrapbooking. Plant a garden, or weed the one you have. Hose off the car. Do a crossword puzzle. Go for a walk with your dog. Meet your neighbors. Do ANYTHING but eat when you're coping with an emotion instead of true hunger.

Get Out of Dodge. A number of my patients have rooms that are strictly off-limits for food, like their bedrooms. This not only keeps your house clear of crumbs, but it also means that there's always a safe haven to retreat to when the siren call of the cookie jar gets too hard to ignore.

One patient goes and sits in a particular armchair with a large glass of water until the craving passes. Another has set up a corner of her den with a couple of big pillows and pictures of her family; when she's having a hard time, she does some yoga or meditates there. Because she never eats there, it's not a place that's associated with food.

Sometimes just designating an area "food-free" is enough to make a significant difference. One of my patients had set up a real bachelor lair in his basement, complete with pool table, widescreen—and fridge. He attributes his ability to make the final forty-pound push to his goal weight to one thing: getting rid of that fridge.

FOOD ADDICTION

"An alcoholic can stop drinking, stop going to bars, stop hanging around people who drink. A drug addict can stop doing drugs. But I have to eat to live, which means I have to face my demons at every single meal."

Food addiction is a compulsion, much like the one that drives people who are addicted to drugs or alcohol. And surgery is not always a match for it; food addiction is absolutely something you need to be treated for, whether you've had the surgery or not.

Are you addicted to food? If you are addicted to food, is it your only addiction? Have you had others in the past? Are you currently practicing other addictions? What have you done thus far in your life to deal with your addictions? Are you open to learning healthy ways to deal with them? These are all questions that a counselor trained in food addiction will ask you if you suspect that you are addicted to food.

Many of my patients join recovery groups such as Overeaters Anonymous that take the twelve-step approach to this problem. Psychiatric drugs and counseling can also help you to break the cycle; ask your doctor for a referral to someone who can help.

After the Honeymoon:
A Year Out and Beyond

Most people who've had the bypass lose the majority of their weight in the first year to year and a half after surgery. For people who've had the band, weight loss is slower, often continuing for up to two years or longer. With both (although more with bypass than the band), what we usually see is that people reach their lowest weight, gain a little back (we often refer to this as "bounce-back weight"), and then level off.

Long-term success, as I'm sure you've gathered already, has everything to do with your compliance with your new lifestyle. But the long-term prognosis, both in my own practice and in the published studies, is very good indeed. If you continue to do the basics, you will be successful.

Reaching Goal

I like to be involved in determining a patient's goal weight with them, and I'd suggest that you ask your own surgeon's opinion about your goal weight, too. Don't set yourself up for failure by setting your goal weight too low. Just because you weighed 130 pounds in high school doesn't mean it's an appropriate weight for you now—or an achievable one.

I'm happy as long as my patients cross the BMI threshold for a nonobese weight (less than 30), because that's when we know that significant co-morbidities begin. Ideally they will push through to a BMI of 25, but it's not essential; after all, we know that health improves even with a small weight loss—as little as 10 percent.

When you get to goal, I hope you'll make a fuss over yourself. Throw a party, send out an e-mail blast with an updated photo of yourself, take a trip. You've accomplished something tremendous, and you deserve all the praise and encouragement you get.

Of course, my priority is to see you maintain your success, and I can tell you that keeping your forward momentum and maintaining your loss will be easier if you've learned good food habits and if you've managed to harness your emotional eating.

> **Remember that reaching goal does not mean that you can start eating anything you want.**

It also does not mean that you can stop taking your vitamin supplements or showing up for your regularly scheduled doctor's appointments. These things are still hugely important. Patients have told me that when they achieve their goal weight they no longer want anything to do with the obese person they were before—including sitting in the waiting room of their weight-loss surgeon's office. But as they always say at our clinic, "Weight loss is not a destination but a journey."

And don't ignore abdominal pain! I've had people come to me five years out with a problem; never forget that a postoperative complication can happen anytime.

Regaining the Weight

"I saw a three-pound gain, and I freaked out. I mean, I freaked out! And then I realized—this is disordered eating, too."

"After my divorce, I started eating again, and gaining. Maybe I was angry at my new body for being the reason my husband and I broke up, although, of course, it's not why we didn't work. But I wish I'd gotten some help; it's been much harder losing all this weight the second time."

A lot of weight-loss surgery patients are very worried about regaining their weight, and rightfully so. I'm happy to say that serious weight gain happens to very few of our patients, and I think it has to do with the kind of aftercare that we provide. Support is one of the most important factors in long-term success. When you sense yourself getting in trouble, it's time to reach out and ask for help.

Have a weight cap. When a patient of mine settles in to their final weight, I suggest that they weigh themselves weekly, at roughly the same time of day (before breakfast is good).

If the scale shows more than five pounds over their goal weight for two weeks in a row, it's time to take action. Don't panic; simply go back to the basics. Make sure you're making healthy food choices, focusing on lean proteins and small portions of complex carbohydrates. Go back to keeping a food journal if you've stopped. Increase your water intake, and ramp things up in the exercise department. Your support group can be an invaluable resource now; take advantage of it.

If you hit ten pounds over your goal weight, it's time to call your surgeon's practice. I know that this can be hard, *but you must do it.* You may feel embarrassed or ashamed, but there's no reason for it: all you need is help refocusing on your goals. If you're working with a good bariatric surgeon, he or she will be as interested in your long-term support and aftercare as when doing surgery on you in the first place. Your success is their success.

I know I've gone on and on about how this surgery is just a tool—and it is. But the fact is that people *do* keep the weight off after surgery. Long-term studies on the bypass and the band show that a significant percentage of the weight—50 to 70 percent in bypass patients—is kept off for many years. It *does* work. Don't prepare yourself for failure—the way you have with diets in the past—instead, get ready to rejoice in your success.

||||||||||||||||||||||||||||||||||||||||||||||||||||||||||||||||||||||||||||

CHAPTER FOURTEEN

Exercise

The Wonder Drug

"My daily walks have become absolutely essential 'me time.' They're a moment of solitude away from my job, my kids, e-mail, the phone—there's nothing to do but move and think."

"My best friend and I work out together a few times a week. I feel more connected to her than I have since college."

"Yoga has been an amazing way for me to get to know (and to make friends with!) my brand new body."

Exercise is essential, absolutely essential, after surgery. But not for the reasons you think it is.

Exercise does promote weight loss, especially for bariatric patients in the months following their surgery. After all, the name of the game is to burn more calories than you take in, and when you're taking in very few calories—between 500 and 800, as you will in the early days after your surgery—it doesn't take much to burn a percentage of that.

But exercise, despite everything you've been told your whole life, is actually a pretty inefficient way to burn calories. As I touched on in Chapter 2, the math just doesn't make sense. I'd have to run for *twenty minutes* in order to burn off the calories in the banana I just ate. That's a lot of exercise for a banana! And you can imagine how much I'd have to do in order to burn off a proper meal.

And yet I try to exercise every day, and I want you to make that a goal as well. So why?

Well, first of all, exercise *does* promote weight loss. Societies with a high level of physical activity have much lower obesity rates than ours. In fact, there was a great study that looked at obesity rates in the United States by zip code—and found that the zip codes with the fewest parks and gyms were the ones with the biggest weight problems. You *do* burn calories while you're exercising, and it helps you to build muscle, which burns more calories—even while you're at rest—than fat does. Additionally, exercise raises your basal metabolic rate, which means that you'll burn more calories all day after you've exercised, even if you don't do anything else, than you would if you hadn't.

This metabolism-boosting effect is especially important after surgery. Remember, when you start losing weight, your body naturally tries to slow that process down by slowing your metabolism; exercise speeds it up again. And, unfortunately, not all the weight you lose after surgery is from fat. Some is from muscle; regular exercise has been shown to reduce the amount of muscle you lose as you lose weight.

> Please note: You should not start a strenuous exercise routine for three to six weeks after surgery. Ask your surgeon, and be sure that your family doc or cardiologist has cleared you for an exercise program.

But helping with your weight loss is just one of the things that exercise can do for you. In fact, exercise is such a general all-around health booster that doctors refer to it as the wonder drug. Here's the short list: Exercise measurably improves blood sugar control, reduces triglycerides, increases "good" HDL levels, lowers your blood pressure, reduces abdominal fat, and reduces your risk of heart disease. It strengthens your heart, muscles, bones, and lungs. It boosts your energy level, improves your balance, and makes you look better. And it is strongly protective for all kinds of diseases, including heart disease and cancer; in fact, there is no pharmaceutical on the market that pushes back the biomarkers of aging and disease like exercise.

**Exercise may be the single most effective thing
you can do to make sure that you don't get sick.**

But, maybe most important, *it makes you feel good*. Austin Davis, a fitness educator to the bariatric community and beyond, goes so far as to call himself a happy-drug dealer. (In order to write this chapter, I relied heavily on Austin, who owns the fitness company FitandFunny.net. He is both very fit and very funny—and if you know him from *Big Medicine* or from his wildly popular seminars, it'll be very clear to you which parts he contributed.)

Austin puts it this way: "One of the reasons that people eat too much is because food acts like a drug that triggers happy receptors in their brains. It's also why we see people cross-addict after surgery—because their brains are looking for the happy fix they used to get from food in shopping, or gambling, or drinking, or sex. Exercise is an addict's secret weapon. Not only does it make the rest of your body healthy—undoing some of the damage you've done to it over the years—but it gives you a cheap, safe 'happy fix.'"

And he's right. Exercise has been scientifically proven to affect mood; it does, in fact, hit exactly the same receptors in the brain that are triggered when we buy something new or eat a piece of chocolate cake.

And exercise also does something else of tremendous value to the obese and the formerly obese—it helps to bring your mind back in line with your body. Let's face it: When you're severely overweight, you spend a lot of time trying to ignore everything from your neck down. Your body isn't a source of pride or something you admire. Is it any wonder that you don't take very good care of it? Austin likes to quote Ronald Reagan: "Nobody washes a rental car." You might be proud of your smile or your brains, but very few people suffering from obesity can point to a part of their body that they really *love*.

All that changes when you start exercising. Exercise helps your body to work better—and when your body works better, you tend to take better care of it. Exercise gives you what Austin calls "a sense of stewardship"—and that not only helps with confidence, but it makes it easier to make the good choices you need to make in order to promote your success.

Exercise Is for *Everyone*

"My doctor told me that water aerobics was the best exercise for me. I know women who wear a size 10 who wouldn't be seen dead in a bathing suit. You think it's easier when you're a size 38?"

"I went to a gym, but there wasn't anything I could do! I couldn't fit on the bikes, I was scared I would break the treadmill, and I can't lie on my back to do ab exercises without having breathing problems. It wasn't that I didn't want to work out; I didn't know what I could do."

I want you to know, right off the bat, that I'm sensitive to the issues that obese people deal with when they exercise.

When you're very large, just holding yourself up long enough to take a shower can be impossible. "Before surgery, I could no sooner have walked to the mailbox than to the moon," one patient told me. The friction of excess flesh can make exercise uncomfortable and even painful, and the body-conscious atmosphere at most gyms—never mind the pool—can be deeply upsetting.

Patients suffering from obesity are also at higher risk for exercise-related injury. Done incorrectly, working out can increase your risk for joint problems, bring on a dangerously elevated heart rate, and result in injuries from a fall. Because body biomechanics are different, you may suffer from poor balance.

But—as Austin likes to say—all of those are obstacles, not barriers. In truth:

Everyone can exercise—
no matter how big you are or how long it's been.

There are lots of things you can do to improve your fitness, even if you're bedridden, and there are lots of ways to work around your physical issues, whatever they might be. And you don't have to go to a gym if you don't feel comfortable; you can just work out at home.

We'll talk about all these issues in great detail in this chapter, but I'll

tell you right now: These aren't going to be your probl
to success—and this is true for everyone—is your
goal in this chapter is not only to give you what
life-extending, happy-making wonder drug in a pe
but also the mental tools you need to take advantage of it.

The Importance of Goals

There is nothing more crucially important when starting a fitness program than to set goals for yourself. If you don't know where you're going, then how are you supposed to get there? If you don't make a commitment to something, then how will you know if you're getting off course?

The first time Austin meets with a new client, he hands them a small spiral-bound notebook and tells them to write the following phrase at the top of the first page: "Are my actions consistent with my goals?" He asks them to write the date, then a short list of specific and achievable goals beneath it. And then he tells them to do that same thing *every single day*.

This is the one thing that each of his clients points to when looking to credit their success. Not the workouts or Austin's winning personality but the act of writing their goals down, every single day.

Austin says:

Habits that aren't reinforced are easily lost.

When times are good, you're not going to have trouble staying on the program. But when times are tough, you're going to want to retreat to "comfort" behaviors, like choosing an old movie or a favorite novel over the gym. That's why you have goals, and that's why I recommend that you write them down every day. Your goals mean that you always have something to return to—even when you fall off the wagon or fail in some other way. That's why they are so important. We need to break you of the ic dieter's mind-set: "I failed, so forget it." In life (and certainly in ess), everyone fails some of the time. The people who ultimately suc-eed are the people who say, "Wow, *that* was incredibly lame, but I'm not going to miss my scheduled workout tomorrow." Having specific goals—and reinforcing them for yourself every single day—helps you do that.

Your goals will necessarily evolve—ideally, as you achieve them! And they have to be realistic for you. Although some of the goals that you'll write in your notebook will be exercise oriented—"I want to be able to run a mile" or "I want to be able to go for a walk on the beach with my kids," they don't have to be. You can integrate everything you want for the future—whether that's success at your job, in your relationships, or any-where else.

We're going to talk now about the three big rules of exercise, as well as the three levels of exercise. You may be surprised by what you read, but I hope you'll stick with these principles, because they work.

Rule #1: First, Do No Harm

"First, do no harm" is part of the Hippocratic oath—the vow that doc-tors take when they become doctors—and it's something you should agree to as you begin your exercise program. There is absolutely no point in working out if you're going to sideline yourself and lose all the benefits you've gained. The point is to get you fitter—not injured.

Exercise shouldn't hurt.

Well, that's not entirely true. You'll have moments of muscle soreness and fatigue; there will be times when your lungs burn and your heart beats faster than you're used to. Those things are necessary on your way to be-coming a fitter, stronger person. But you should never feel real pain, and here are some guidelines to help:

Start slow! At the very beginning, you may not be fit enough to do much of anything at all. But you don't have to sign up for an ultramarathon—just do *something*. Walk to the mailbox. If that's too far, walk around the room. If that's too much, walk from one end of the room to another—or from the couch to the coffee table.

You might feel very motivated by the thought of this new program. That's great—but don't take it as a reason to go out for a run. If you haven't worked out in a long time, it's downright unsafe to throw yourself into a hard-core regime, and it will make it much harder to stay consistent, which is our real goal.

You might feel discouraged in these early days by how little you can do. Just remember: *This isn't it*. It's the first step in a long journey. If you keep doing something, I personally guarantee that you will look back at where you started with real pride at how far you've come.

In the meantime, let's see what we can do to remove some of the obstacles preventing you from exercising comfortably so that you're as comfortable as you can be.

Fight friction. If you're still losing, your excess flesh can bounce around and make exercise uncomfortable; later, when you've lost more weight, you may find yourself coping with extra skin.

Chafing hurts! One solution is to use antichafing gels such as BodyGlide and Sportsslick. These were developed for long-distance runners, but my patients love them. You can order them online or buy them in a sporting goods store.

What you wear also plays a role. If you feel most comfortable in baggy workout clothes, fine—but do wear something more supportive underneath. This will prevent the movement and friction that make you so uncomfortable. Women (of all sizes) can save themselves a lot of pain by making sure they have an extremely supportive sports bra when they exercise. Overweight men often carry their weight in their chest and belly, so they may want to consider wearing a spandex shirt or tank top underneath their T-shirt.

A number of companies specialize in supportive undergarments (sometimes called compression wear), including:

Enell: Enell.com. This company makes sports bras up to size 50DDD to 52DD and will custom-make a bra in any larger size. Women rave about them (even Oprah)—they're very supportive, even for very large-breasted women. They also make a custom-fit support vest for men.

Morris Designs: MorrisDesigns.com. This company specializes in compression garments for men and for women.

ContourMD: ContourMD.com. This company specializes in postsurgical compression garments and has a bariatric section.

Stay hydrated. Weight-loss surgery patients get dehydrated easily because their small stomachs make it harder for them to take in adequate fluids. Never work out without a source of water nearby, and make sure you're drinking lots of it—before, during, and after your workout.

Invest in good shoes. Good exercise shoes are a necessity, not a luxury. That's true for everyone, but it's especially true for overweight people.

Sneaker technology is a big business, and the selection can be a little overwhelming. Everyone's feet are different; don't be surprised if even a top-of-the-line shoe feels uncomfortable. The wrong fit can actually cause injury, so make sure you've got the right pair for you. You'll know you've found them because they'll feel good right off the bat. If they're not comfortable in that first step, they won't ever be comfortable; keep shopping until you've found a better match.

And you'll have to replace your sneakers often, as often as a marathon runner does. Being obese takes a real toll on your shoes—just like it does on your joints. I'd estimate that you'll need a new pair of workout shoes every six months; keep an eye on the soles for signs of wear. There will be other signs, too: If you've been working out without pain for a few months and suddenly start getting soreness in your knees or ankles, that's another indication that you've pushed your shoes too far. Ignore these warnings at your peril!

Warm up—and cool down. Leave five or ten minutes before and after your workouts for warm-up and cool-down. The warm-up gets your heart and muscles ready for what you're about to ask of them by increasing blood flow—and it gets your brain ready, too. Use gentle movements (see the box on the next page for an example of some things you can do) to get your engines revving, and don't hit the locker room before your breathing and heart rate have returned to normal.

HELLO, BODY!

We've all been startled into wakefulness by the screech of an alarm clock. It's not a very relaxing way to start the day, which is why some newer alarms wake you up by slowly increasing in volume or with a gently blinking light.

This exercise is the equivalent of those alarms. It's not a fitness exercise, per se—although it may feel like it is for some people just starting out. (You can also do a version of it from a seated position.) I like to do this before I begin working out, but I also use it as a way to clear my head when I've been driving a long distance or sitting in front of a computer screen too long. It's a gentle way to wake up your body and for you to reconnect with it.

Please note: All of these movements should be done without strain.

Stand in a comfortable, wide stance. Let your arms hang loosely at your sides. Take a deep breath in, and exhale. Turn your head slowly to one side, so that you're looking over your shoulder. Keep breathing, making note of any tension you feel. Hold there, and then slowly move your head so that you're looking in the other direction. Look up, and look down. Tilt your head so that your ear faces your shoulder, and then repeat on the other side. When your neck feels warmed up, make gentle circles with your head, all the way around, and then reverse the direction.

Roll your shoulders slowly, first front, then back. Make the movements complete, so that you really feel the muscles in your chest and back. Hunch your shoulders forward, as if you were trying to touch them together in front of you, and then push your chest out, arching your back.

Moving down your body, slowly move your hips from one side to the other. If you can, make a wide circle with them, first in one direction and then the other. Bend your knees gently, and straighten your legs a few times, warming up your knees. Hang over at your waist, letting your arms dangle like a rag doll. You're not trying to touch your toes; you're simply waking up the back of your legs and your lower back. Finally, stand on one leg (hold onto something if your balance is unsure) and roll your ankles, first one way, and then the other.

Now that you've woken up the big muscle groups, take a minute or two to move your body in whatever way feels good to you. Roll your neck and shoulders, swing your arms gently, and bounce on your toes. Let your body tell you what it needs.

Rule #2: Consistency, Consistency, Consistency

You've probably heard the Woody Allen quote that 90 percent of life is just showing up. Well, that's never truer than when it applies to exercise.

Now, you're going to have to do quite a bit more than simply show up; nothing's going to happen if you're just sitting around in your sweatpants. But if you're trying to establish new habits, it is better for you to show up and do a little bit less than what you're completely capable of than for you to blow off your workout altogether, promising to do something with more intensity tomorrow. Too often that tomorrow never comes, and one day off from your program becomes months.

So I'd like you to commit to something that absolutely everyone can do if they choose: Work out for just ten minutes, three times a week.

A half hour a week—that's it!

I know, I know—you're about to tell me that the American College of Sports Medicine recommends a minimum of an hour's hard exercise every day. But the majority of Americans—70 percent of them, by some estimates—don't get any exercise at all. If you can go from nothing at all to half an hour a week, that's a truly significant improvement.

Austin says:

It's not your weight that matters; it's your habits.

That's it. That's the first level of exercise: ten minutes, three times a week.

Now, you have to schedule those workouts—and you have to keep those appointments with yourself. You see, something interesting happens when you make a consistent commitment to a little bit of exercise. You do three sessions of just ten minutes over the course of the week, and you start to think, "Well, that wasn't so bad." And the next time you run out of steam in front of your computer, you find yourself on your feet and moving around. Or your coworker compliments you on how diligent you've been about your workouts, and you like the feeling—so the next time you go out for a ten-minute bout, you find yourself staying out for fifteen minutes, and then twenty. Or you do those ten-minute spurts every day.

You know what? Twenty minutes, three times a week, is the second level of exercise. So without even realizing it, you're already making progress. Slowly, you get into shape. You start to relish the way your body feels when it's in motion, and you start to crave the way it feels when you stop. The third level of exercise is four or five times a week, for half an hour. That's what I do, and it's what most of my patients a year or more out aim for. You'll get there, too!

And by always keeping that ten-minute, three-times-a-week workout as your minimum, you give yourself a very workable baseline—one that you can maintain even when life gets crazy. I'm not unrealistic; there are going to be times when you're doing all you can to keep up with whatever else is going on in your life. But, no matter how all-consuming the other things in your life are, *you can always do ten minutes, three times a week.* And when your mom gets better, or your kid no longer requires constant supervision, or your book deadline has passed, it will be a lot easier to get back into the swing of your workouts. Because you're not starting from zero—you're starting from your baseline of three ten-minute sessions a week.

AUSTIN'S TELEVISION WORKOUT

Let's say you watch three hours of television a week. (The average American watches more like twenty-eight hours a week, according to the Nielsen company; even if you watch a quarter of that, you'll have plenty of time for this workout.) There are about twenty minutes of commercials during the average show. So if you work out just during the commercials and during just one show, three times a week, you've done an hour of exercise by the time the week is over. That's the second level of exercise—and all while you're watching television.

Would I rather you turn the tube off? Yes, of course; this isn't an ideal workout. But the first step in being successful is to get it done, and if working out this way will get you to work out, then I'm all for it.

Rule #3: Recognize a Relapse

It's very easy to get into an "all or nothing" mind-set—it's something you learned in your bad-old dieting days. But even though you might be in a slightly better place with food now because of the surgery, it's easy to revert to those old patterns when we're talking about fitness.

Here's what that looks like. When you're working out, you work out like nobody's business. But when you stop, you just STOP. There isn't a whole lot of middle ground. That's why it's so enormously important—no matter what you do—to get your three workouts in. At just ten minutes a pop, there's really no excuse. And doing this for a few months will really help you to reprogram your mind-set.

But when you do fall off—and you *will* fall off—how do you put on the brakes before you've gone six months without lacing up your sneakers? You have to be able to identify a relapse.

Identifying a relapse:

- Have you missed more than two scheduled sessions?

- Has it been more than a week since you exercised?

- Have you gained weight? (Anything more than five or ten pounds is a warning flag.)

If the answer to any of these questions—not all of them, but *any* of them—is yes, then you're relapsing. No matter how many good excuses you have (and you will have them), that's the simple truth. But the diagnosis is the first step to getting you back on track. Next, you have to answer the following questions:

Did you stop because you got hurt? If your hip hurts, your knee hurts, your ankles are killing you, your low back won't go—then you did the right thing when you stopped exercising. Pain is nature's way of telling you to stop what you're doing. Forget about all that nonsense about "playing through pain"—there's only a more serious injury at the end of that rainbow. Carrying too much weight is hard on the body, particularly on the joints, and many injuries only start popping up once you start losing the weight.

If something starts to hurt, the first thing you should do is *go see a doctor*. Get some relief for that pain.

The next thing you have to do is find a way to exercise around the pain.

**While you shouldn't ever exercise *through* pain,
you can—and must—exercise *around* it.**

There are as many modifications for an exercise routine as there are injuries. If your knees are bugging you, then you should stop walking. But there's no reason you can't do something else, something that builds strength and endurance. As you'll see a little later, there are tons of exercises you can do while sitting down; do them on a stability ball. Use the hula hoop on your upper body. Borrow a neighbor's pool. Just find something, and do it—for a minimum of ten minutes, three times a week.

If you're not hurt but stopped for another reason, can you commit to three ten-minute workouts a week? If the answer to that question is no, then it's likely that you're bumping up against some mental resistance. *Everyone* can find three ten-minute sessions a week. Everyone. (That ten minutes can even be cumulative, over the course of the day!) So if you "can't"—then you've made a decision to move away from your goals instead of toward them. This means it's time for a reevaluation. Have you set goals that are too difficult to achieve, or are they wrong for you? Is there something else going on, some form of self-sabotage or fear that's preventing you from doing what you need to do?

This is a great time to reach out and get some support. Talk to the members of your support group: Can a fitness expert come to speak to the group? Is there someone in the group who will work out with you until you get back on track, or do they work with a personal trainer who'd do a session or two with you? Will someone call you on the morning of your scheduled workout to make you accountable?

Reach out, get a strategy in gear, and get back into it.

Austin says:

There are only two motivations in life: avoiding pain and gaining pleasure. Are your pleasures causing you pain? Or is the pain you are avoiding actually the very thing to bring you pleasure?

Did you get bored? It's easy to get locked into doing one thing. "This is the thing that works for me," you think to yourself. But it's not a great idea. Doing the same exercises over and over leaves you open to overuse injuries, for one thing. Plus, your muscles get used to doing the same thing over and over again, which means you're not using your workout time as efficiently as you should.

And it *is* boring: If you spend half an hour on a treadmill four times a week, eventually you're going to start feeling like a hamster on a wheel. So do something different. Learn to social dance, go roller-skating, try a hula-hoop—it doesn't matter what it is, as long as you're moving.

The Motivation Problem: What's in Your Bag of Tricks?

"I hate exercising!" you say.

Here's a news flash for you: Everybody hates exercise some of the time. That guy training for the triathlon in the freezing-cold rain at 5:30 in the morning? He'd rather be hitting the snooze button, too. But he knows two things. First of all, he knows he's going to feel like a million bucks when he's done—and that's terrific positive reinforcement every time. And he knows that he made a commitment to his training. You made a similar commitment when you had surgery. So keep it—and know that you'll be reaping the rewards of that happy drug all day long.

You don't have to like it.
You just have to do it.

Mary Jo—an endurance runner, by the way—says that the only difference between people who are out of shape and athletes is that athletes
have better tricks at their disposal. On a cold morning, an athlete looks out
the window and says, "I'll just go for five minutes, and if it's totally awful, I
can come home again." Of course, once she's out there, hitting her stride
and getting warmed up, there's no chance she's turning around.

Distractions aren't necessarily a bad thing, as long as you're getting your
workout done. I know one marathoner who uses her running partner as a
television. They each watch different reality shows over the course of the
week, and then tell each other the plots—in incredibly intricate detail—
during their long weekend runs. Silly? Maybe. "Anything to get through
mile nineteen," she tells me. Do whatever you have to do to get yourself to
start. Once you've begun, you'll easily see how the snowball rolls down-
hill.

Music can be a big motivator, and one that's too often overlooked. There's
a reason that professional sports teams get fired up by listening to an inspirational song together in the locker room before they head out to compete. The
right music can get your emotions charged and your blood pumping. And it
can help you later, when your energy flags. The steady beat can help your
rhythm, too. Listen to what inspires you—and don't be surprised if the music you like to listen to while you're working out isn't the same kind of music
you like to listen to over dinner!

When all else fails, go back to your goals. What do you want? And do
the choices you're making support your goals?

Focus on Functional Fitness

Let's talk now about some exercises that you can do—no matter who
you are or what kind of shape you're in. Before we begin, I'd like to introduce one more concept that will help you as you begin to design your
workout: functional fitness.

Functional fitness is, very simply, the idea that you're training at the
gym in order to perform better outside of it. The squat, for instance, is the
perfect example of a functional exercise. What do you do in life more than
squat? You squat every time you sit down on the couch or the toilet—and
you squat every time you get up. What's walking up the stairs, if not a
one-legged squat? Working on building the muscles you need to do that

exercise efficiently won't just give you great legs but will benefit you many, many times a day.

I love it when my patients come in and tell me they've noticed things getting easier since they started working out. "My briefcase feels empty," one told me. "I hung out in the pool for two hours with my kids and never felt tired," said another.

Use the idea of functional fitness to help you create goals for your workouts. What would you like to be able to do in your life that would require you to be in better shape?

Let me give you an example. One of Austin's clients mentioned to him during their introductory session that her daughter was six months pregnant. He saw the opportunity and leapt on it. "That means that in just a few months, you're going to be spending a lot of time with a ten-pound weight in your arms. Wouldn't it be nice if you could actually manage that ten-pound weight? What kinds of things will you want to do with it? Will you want to hoist it up onto your shoulder, walk around with it until it dozes off, swing it around to make it giggle? Will you want to be able to hold it in one arm while you prepare a bottle with another, or answer the phone?"

Knowing that her work with the weights and the medicine ball was going to facilitate something important in her life—helping her daughter at an overwhelming time, and bonding with her new granddaughter—gave that client's workouts new purpose.

If you can't walk, you can't walk your daughter down the aisle on her wedding day. If you can't lift a suitcase, you can't travel. If you can't do a squat, you can't stand up to give a standing ovation. So take a moment to write down the things in your life for which you'd like to get fit and strong.

Keep these goals in mind as you're putting together a workout for yourself. What types of exercises would help you to "train" for these activities? (This list is a terrific thing to share with a personal trainer, by the way.)

I encourage people to focus on three areas: strength (so you can lift things, including your own body weight), flexibility (so you can bend down to get something without feeling creaky), and endurance (so the activities of daily life don't exhaust you). A program that combines some type of resistance training with yoga and a cardio workout, for example, would be ideal.

Exercise Suggestions

Stretching. Although you may think about stretching as something you do before or after a workout, for a person suffering from obesity, a stretching session can provide a low-impact way to move each part of your body. I personally don't like the way it feels to stretch cold muscles; I prefer to stretch after I've warmed up a little.

When you stretch:

- Hold the stretch for ten seconds if you can.

- *Don't* bounce.

- *Don't* go so far that it hurts. You should feel something—but that something shouldn't be pain.

- *Don't* get competitive about it. Some people are naturally flexible; others aren't. Some parts of your body may be comparatively flexible, while others are very stiff. And you'll notice that you're tighter some days than others—sometimes even that you're tighter on one side! Stay in touch with what your body is telling you and respect your own limits.

- Breathe! There is a temptation to hold your breath while you're stretching, but it's counterproductive. Instead, try pushing a little farther into the stretch as you relax with your exhale.

There are hundreds of low-impact stretching and yoga DVDs out there. Try one, and see how different your body begins to feel after a few sessions.

Walking. In the early days after surgery, you're going to be walking.

I like to recommend walking because you can do it anywhere (which is great for people who travel a lot or who tend to feel self-conscious at the gym). You can walk in your neighborhood, at a school track, in the park, or at the mall. You don't need a lot of fancy equipment, except for very good, shock-absorbent shoes.

When I see patients who are very overweight or who haven't worked out in a while, I ask them first just to increase the number of steps they take in a day. There are a number of good and very inexpensive pedometers on the market. Get used to clipping one on your belt. Every day log how many steps you've taken, and try to increase it by 10 percent the next day. It's not hard to do over the course of a normal day: Just park at the back of the lot or take the stairs. Put away the remote control and change the channels by hand; you'll be surprised! For an added bonus, move around your house during the commercial breaks.

I have patients who go for a four- or five-minute walk around their office every hour on the hour. One patient has gotten into the habit of getting off the train one stop before she needs to, either on her way in to work or on her way home. Her goal, by the end of the summer, is to be doing it both ways. And when she gets a little more fit, I hope she'll consider adding a weighted vest.

Use the stairs. Going up the stairs is terrific exercise; it builds a lot of strength in your lower body, and there's cardiovascular benefit as well. Spend your ten minutes going up and down the stairs, and you'll really feel it.

Remember, too: Exercise is cumulative. If you walk up and down the stairs instead of using the elevator at work, for instance, those minutes can really add up. One minute when you come in every morning, two minutes when you go out and come back from lunch, two minutes when you go to visit your buddy in accounting, one minute on your way out—that's half your session right there.

Rebounder. Minitrampolines are wonderful. Don't worry; you're not going to be jumping—not unless you want to. But in the same way that walking on the beach is harder and works more muscles than walking on concrete does, marching in place on the rebounder takes walking to the next level. Best of all, it cushions your joints very effectively, making it a good, low-impact choice for people who traditionally have trouble with their knees. (Although you'll want to avoid it if you have ankle problems.)

If you want to increase your workout, you can move your arms while you're marching. Start with both arms in front of your chest, and push one arm—and then the other—up into the air with every step you take, as if you were climbing a ladder. Eventually you can do this with hand weights.

AUSTIN SAYS:

Buy Good Quality Equipment Used! There's no need to spend a lot on new exercise equipment or to buy lower-quality stuff new. If you go to ten garage sales in a weekend, you're pretty much guaranteed to find everything you could possibly want, and for just a few bucks. If not, try craigslist.com in your city; you'll find lots of barely used, high-quality equipment for a song.

And if you get bored with it (or find that you've bought something that doesn't work for you), don't let it become a clothes-hanger in the corner of your bedroom. Get it out of your house by reposting it, and make room for something new.

Exercise ball. You've probably seen these big, brightly colored balls on television. They're great for strengthening the core and back, but they also help with balance. Just sitting on an exercise ball is hard work for your abs and back and thighs; use one instead of a chair while you watch TV or surf the Internet, and you'll see what I mean!

There are lots of exercises specific to the ball, and you can also use the ball as a kind of exercise bench, resting your back on it while you do a chest press, for instance. You can also use a ball to build your upper body; they're light, but they require that you use a lot of different muscles to stabilize them.

BallDynamics.com sells balls that are burst resistant to well over 1,000 pounds. Make sure to use the charts to pick the appropriate size for your height; the taller you are, the bigger a ball you'll need.

Weight training. Perhaps the phrase *weight training* calls to mind a massive bodybuilder, straining to lift a barbell above his head. It's time to refresh that image! In fact, people of all shapes and sizes can benefit from training with weights—and weights are available in all sizes, some as light as two pounds.

I think a set of dumbbells in a few different weights is a great investment; they're cheap, and they don't take up any space. When you get a little more fit, you can also incorporate them into your cardio routine.

Basic Weight Workout

The workout I've given you here will take just minutes to do, and it can be very easily modified. If you have limited mobility, do it sitting down on a sturdy stool or on an exercise ball. Later you can do it standing up; eventually you can do many of these exercises from a squatting or a lunge position.

If working with even the lightest weights is too much, then simply use your own body weight for the first two weeks.

Note: It's essential to do these exercises correctly and with proper form so that you see the results you want and don't get hurt. If you've never used weights before, ask a pro at your gym for guidance, rent a weight-training DVD, or search for videos on YouTube, where a lot of trainers have put up weight-training guides. Once you know how to use them, use a mirror to ensure that you're using proper form.

Lifting weights properly means:

- Your torso should stay straight and still during arm and leg exercises—the only thing that should be moving is the muscle you're using to do the exercise.

- You don't rely on your body's momentum to raise the weights, and you don't swing them around.

- Your knees and elbows should be "soft"—not bent, but not ramrod straight and hyperextended, either. Feet should be hip-width apart.

- You should *never* feel a sharp pain or pull; if you do, stop immediately and consider whether a lighter weight is a better choice for you.

- You keep your hands, wrists, and forearms in a straight line during arm exercises. You don't want to bend your wrists to help move the weight, as this can cause a repetitive stress injury.

- You don't forget to breathe!

Basic Exercises

If you can do more than fifteen or twenty repetitions with a particular weight, it's time to consider using something a little heavier.

Side and front raises. Keeping your wrists straight, raise your arms to the sides, never going higher than your shoulders. Return your arms to your sides. Next, raise your arms to the front, again stopping when you reach shoulder height. Return your arms to your sides.

Shoulder press. Starting with the weights at shoulder height, elbows bent, push the weights over your head up to the ceiling. Lower them slowly.

Bicep curl. Extend your arms down by your sides, facing outward. Keeping your elbows close to your body, bend them, bringing the weights up toward your shoulders. Lower slowly.

Gentle twist. Hold your arms by your sides, and bend your elbows so that the weights are right in front of your chest. Keeping your hips facing front, gently twist your body to the right, and then to the left. The weights should stay even the whole time.

Squats. Keeping your feet parallel and pushing your rear end back, bend your knees as if to sit on an invisible stool. (Your knees should *never* go in front of your toes.) Straighten your legs and return to a standing position. After one set, turn your toes out slightly in order to work your inner thighs. Holding your hand weights while you do this exercise will increase your workout.

You can even work out your lower body from a seated position on a sturdy stool. While sitting down:

"Walk" in place. Pull in your tummy, and raise your knees as if you were walking.

Slide one foot out so that your leg is extended, and then pull it back in and push the other foot out.

With your knees bent and feet flat on the floor, slide your feet out so that your thighs form a V. Slide them back in again.

Pulling your belly in, extend one leg so that it's shooting straight out from your hip. Put it down, then extend the other leg. If you can, hold the extension for five seconds.

Bend your elbows by your sides and hold your weights there while you do this—put them down if this is too much. When you get stronger, adding adjustable ankle weights will improve this workout.

"WON'T WEIGHT TRAINING MAKE ME BIGGER?"

I've been asked this question more times than I can count, especially by women who are—quite naturally—looking to avoid anything that bulks them up, even if that bulk is muscle and not fat.

The answer is: Not really. Muscle does weigh a little more than fat, and it can add inches. But you really have to be moving some pretty serious weight for that to happen, as any teenage kid trying to put on muscle will tell you. And whatever you gain in bulk from weight training is more than offset by how much better it makes you look.

"OUCH! I'M SORE!"

Slight muscle soreness is a fact of life when you exercise, but it can be quite intense when you start after a period of time away. You may also notice that you're more sore two days after a workout than you are right after. That's called delayed onset muscle soreness, and it's perfectly normal.

I personally like the feeling; it makes me feel like I've done something! But there are a few things you can do to speed healing. If your bathtub will accommodate you comfortably, take baths as hot as you can tolerate them. Add two cups of Epsom salts, and sit in there for as long as you can. Drink water while you're soaking, and get out immediately if you feel you're getting dizzy or light-headed.

The temptation will be to recover by parking yourself on the couch, but getting blood to your sore muscles will help them to recover faster. So move! Stretching does help; do a little while you watch television. Going for a short walk—even just ten minutes—will get blood moving into the muscles.

Remember: NO NSAIDs! If you've had a bypass, these anti-inflammatory drugs are off-limits to you for the rest of your life. (Tylenol is still okay.)

Pedal exercisers. There are several portable pedal exercisers available. They are convenient because you can use them with any chair, unlike a recumbent bike. I especially like these for my patients because they can be used for both the upper and lower body. If your knee is bothering you, you can still get your cardio—just put the exerciser on a desk and do it with your arms!

Bodyblade. This is one of Austin's favorites for bariatric clients; in fact, you may have seen him use it with Allan on *Big Medicine*. It's an odd looking thing—a flexible board with a handgrip in the middle—but it's a great way to build muscle and to stabilize the core muscles that carry you through life, while raising your heart rate. It can even be done from a bed: Austin calls it his secret weapon with limited mobility or bed-bound patients. You can find it, along with instructions for using it, at Bodyblade.com.

Hula hoop. Another one of Austin's secret weapons. The great thing about the hula hoop is that it's fun—you hardly notice that you're getting your heart rate up. But the other thing that's great about it is that you move it around your body. If you can't stand up, you can circle it around one arm and then the other. If a hula hoop isn't big enough, pick up some flexible PVC tubing at the hardware store and make your own!

Some Other Things to Consider

Use a personal trainer. I can't say enough about the benefits to be gained from working with a good personal trainer. Trainers are knowledgeable, able to personalize a workout for your specific needs, and terrifically motivating.

The problem, of course, is that they're expensive. But you don't need to see a trainer three times a week for it to work; Austin worked with a woman who could only afford to see him once every other month. They spent those sessions crafting a workout that she could do in the intervening time.

If you decide to splurge on a trainer (and I highly recommend that you do, at least a couple of times a year), I'd suggest that you look for one who has experience with overweight people. Ask your surgeon's office for recommendations; they probably have people who work with their patients on a regular basis. You can also ask your support group for recommendations or post the question on an online support forum.

You can also use an online personal trainer, such as Plus One Active—PlusOneActive.com—or Workouts for You—WorkoutsforYou.com.

Join a gym. There are lots of benefits to joining a gym: Gyms have a much wider range of equipment than you'll be able to accumulate at home, including some very cool weight machines. Some people also feel that it's easier to work out if they're not home, staring at a dishwasher that needs emptying and a phone that needs answering.

A lot of my patients have been pleasantly surprised by the wide range of body types at their local gym. "I thought the gym was the place the pretty people went to work out," one patient reported happily, after discovering she wasn't the only new member with 100-plus pounds to lose. It has been my experience that people are at the gym to work out, not to worry about your body and what you're doing. (My female patients report that the all-female atmosphere at women-only gyms such as Curves and Lucille Roberts is helpful for the self-conscious.)

If joining a gym interests you, visit when you're most likely to go. Many gyms are overcrowded on the weekends and after work—but empty in the middle of the day. If you're going to be going during a crowded time, see how long the average wait is for a machine, and if there are sign-up sheets for the cardio machines. Take a careful look around: If the equipment is badly out of date or in poor condition, you can get hurt. Make sure to pick up a class schedule. And take it for a test drive; most gyms will issue a one-day guest pass to prospective members.

Personal training studio. If you feel self-conscious at a gym but want to work out on professional equipment outside of your house, you may want to consider a personal training studio. They are popping up all over, and they often cater to people with special needs. And they often have nutritionists and personal trainers on staff for a more holistic approach to weight loss. Ask around to see if any of the studios near you have experience with the obese or with bariatric patients.

Workout DVDs. I'm a big proponent of these; I work long hours and cannot always get to the gym. With a DVD, I can fit in a workout when I get home or before I leave in the morning.

There are literally thousands of DVDs out there for you to choose from; the reviews on Amazon can steer you in the right direction. Or rent one on Netflix before deciding if you want to add it to your permanent collection.

Austin's new series, available at FitandFunny.net, is specifically designed to bring functional fitness to everybody. Plus-size model Megan
Garcia has a yoga video that many of my patients like to do. And I still
hear great things about oldies-but-goodies Jane Fonda and Richard Sim-
mons.

I do a very intense workout set called P90X. Their motto is "Just push
play, and bring it." I love that: When I get home, I know I can push play
and bring it. The company is Beachbody.com, and I recommend their
Power 90 workout routine for my patients.

Swimming. This is the form of exercise that's most often prescribed
for overweight people. It does keep the weight off your joints, and the water does provide a natural resistance. The problem I have found is that my
patients just don't do it: The self-consciousness factor is simply too great.
The one exception to this seems to be people who have a pool in their own
backyard.

If you do have access to a pool you feel comfortable using, try these
exercises:

Just walking in the shallow end is terrific exercise. Keep your hands
underwater to increase the amount you have to work.

Hold onto the side and lift one leg to the side. Repeat as many times as
you can, and then switch sides.

Squat. Standing in the shallow end, bend your knees and push your
rear end out behind you. (Your knees should never be ahead of your toes.)
Stand back up. Repeat.

Tricep extensions: Keep your arms to the sides and bend them so that
your hands are in front of your waist. Straighten them slowly underwater
so that they're straight by your side.

Stand with your back against the wall and clap your hands underwater.
Keep your fingers closed for extra resistance.

A water aerobics class will give you a lot more good ideas; it's a fun,
low-impact type of workout.

The Law of Diminishing Returns

As you lose weight and are able to exercise more, you'll notice that
something funny happens.

**When it gets easy, you have to do more to see
results.**

If you started out just walking around the house, it's time to go down
the driveway; if you've been walking around your neighborhood, it's time to
walk a little farther—or to jog.

And you are also going to have to keep doing different things in order to
continue to see progress. If you go to the same step class three times a
week, your body is going to get really, really good at doing step; it will, in
other words, become extremely efficient at performing the movements required for you in this class. Unfortunately if you're looking to get in shape,
it means that you're getting a lot less out of that forty minutes of exercise
than you would be getting if you were doing something else.

The best solution is to do three different things—a yoga or Pilates
class, a cardio routine, and strength training, say—for each one of your
training sessions. That way you'll never get efficient enough at any of them
to see diminishing returns. And as you get more fit, your continuing chal-
lenge will be in finding ways to keep your routine fresh. Martial arts, jazz
dance, mountain climbing—these are all ways to exercise.

One tool that has helped a lot of my patients—especially after they've
become more fit—is something called the target heart rate zone. As long
as you achieve and stay in this zone for your workout, it doesn't matter
what you're doing.

Here's why I like it:

- It's individualized. You may look at the Olympic-caliber athlete on
  the treadmill next to yours and think "No way!" But as long as you're
  working in your target heart rate—just as he or she is—then you're
  both getting the workout you need.

- It's dynamic: It changes with you the fitter you get. And you are going to get fitter!

- It's safe: Working within your zone means that you're both working
  out efficiently and safely; by staying within your zone, you're not
  working above it. This is especially important for people who are
  very overweight.

- You don't need any fancy equipment. All you need is your finger, a watch—and your pulse, of course. If math and counting aren't your forte, though, you may want to consider investing in a heart rate monitor; there are a number of good ones available for less than $100.

Finding Your Target Heart Rate Zone

Here's how to find it:

First, subtract your age from the number 220. This number is known as your maximum heart rate. Now we don't want you working at your maximum, but rather between 60 and 70 percent of your heart rate. So let's find those:

$$220 - (\text{your age}) = \text{max heart rate}$$
$$\text{Max Heart Rate} \times .60 = \text{low end of your target heart rate zone}$$
$$\text{Max Heart Rate} \times .70 = \text{high end of your target heart rate zone}$$

But you don't have to count for a minute. Just divide your results by six—and then watch the clock for ten seconds while you're counting.

Please note: If you're still more than fifty pounds overweight, talk to your doctor and make sure you have clearance to exercise; I'd also recommend that you keep your heart rate in the lower end of the zone.

Taking Your Pulse

- You can take your pulse in one of two places: To take your pulse at the wrist, press the pointer and middle fingers of the opposite hand to the area on the inside of the wrist just below the pad of the thumb.

- To take your pulse at the neck, place your fingers over the soft area to one side of the Adam's apple. Do *not* apply pressure to this spot.

Using the target heart rate zone is a great way to maximize your fitness.

You can use it no matter what type of exercise you're doing. As you get stronger and more fit, you'll have to work harder to get into your zone.

‖‖‖‖‖‖‖‖‖

I started this chapter by telling you to take it easy. But I hope you understand that ten minutes, three times a week is really just a starting point. A recent study in the journal *Surgery for Obesity and Related Diseases,* showed that you need to exercise thirty minutes a day, five days a week, if you want to achieve better weight loss than the average surgery patient—and the other benefits of exercise we've discussed.

Walking, working in your garden, and being active at work are certainly better than laying around, but to truly achieve your goals you do need to push yourself. It's much better to work out thirty intense minutes a day than it is to walk for hours and barely break a sweat. And you have to keep your muscles off-balance by changing your workout every few weeks. Not only will doing this keep you interested and looking forward to the gym, but it will shock your muscles into growth.

**Your goals must get more difficult,
and your intensity must build.**

The success that comes from achieving your goals will spill into all areas of your life. So get your goal notebook—and get going!

CHAPTER FIFTEEN

Emotions After Surgery

"This is what I've always wanted. So why do I find myself crying every day?"

"I had no idea how much hurt was hiding underneath all that fat."

"I definitely had low self-esteem, anxiety, and a tendency toward depression before surgery, but I'd never had to cope with those things without food before."

You're losing weight very rapidly and seeing some very profound changes in your body. This can give rise to a lot of complicated feelings. You'll be happy and proud, yes. But you may also experience frustration, depression, guilt, and grief as well. Now that you aren't using food to numb yourself—and the layers of fat aren't there to hide behind anymore—emotions are going to bubble to the surface. Not all of them are going to be entirely pleasant.

This is where all the support we've been talking about comes in. I strongly encourage my patients to talk to someone, and individual counseling with a therapist who has experience with bariatric patients is the best option. In fact, I recommend counseling—even just a few sessions—for all of my patients. Unfortunately, there's still a stigma attached to seeking help during a difficult time (particularly among men in my observation). I'd encourage you to do it anyway; most people undergoing a transformation of this enormity will benefit from a little outside per-spective. A bariatric support group experience, whether live or online, is also pretty much mandatory for my patients. It is tremendously helpful to talk to and listen to people who have walked the same path you're traveling.

In this chapter, I will cover some of the emotional reactions to the sur-gery that we've heard about from our patients over the years in counseling sessions with Mary Jo and in our support groups. The same themes come up often, and I think it's useful to talk about them ahead of time so that you're prepared—and so you won't feel isolated if they come up for you. I've also asked Mary Jo to give examples of some of the exercises she uses with our patients in the support groups to address these issues. (These exercises, while helpful, shouldn't be seen as a replacement for counseling or for the live or online support group experience.)

Please note: This is by no means an exhaustive discussion of the wide range of emotions that people experience after surgery. And if you're con-sidering surgery, don't take the information in this chapter to mean that you automatically will become an emotional wreck! Your quality of life will in fact improve immeasurably, and many of my patients even stop taking antidepressants in the years after surgery. The purpose of this chapter is simply to make you aware of the fact that you don't leave your emotional baggage in the operating room. It is entirely possible—and in-deed very common—to be successful and still to struggle with some of these feelings.

An Increased Sense of Vulnerability

"When I still had the weight, my friends would always worry about me walking around alone late at night. 'Don't you under-stand?' I finally snapped, 'nobody's going to touch me.'"

"I realize now that I used my weight to separate me from the world. I couldn't handle intimacy, and I didn't have to. Now that the weight is gone (most of it, anyhow), it's like—whoa! Where's my buffer?"

As the weight comes off, it may leave you feeling very vulnerable. Your self-image before surgery—as poor as it might have been—was based, at least in part, on your obesity. Being big may have given you a feeling of being invisible—or, conversely, a feeling of power conferred by your size—that you came to rely on, even though it came with tremendous costs.

Now you're no longer obese. And because you're no longer obese, you may no longer be exempt from some of the things—certain responsibilities or types of intimacy—that you were before surgery.

This feeling of vulnerability may creep up on you. A number of my patients have even told me that they now have personal space issues that they'd never experienced before. Before you lost the weight, even someone who was standing very close to you felt like they were farther away, because they *were*—your larger body created a physical buffer zone that is no longer there.

In truth, one of the reasons you had the surgery is because you no longer wanted to look at life from the sidelines. So one of the challenges you'll face now that the weight is off is learning to set physical and emotional boundaries for yourself instead of using your extra flesh to do it.

It can help to explore some of these issues in a journal, with a counselor, or in a support group. What things or experiences make you feel powerful and give you a voice? Can you give examples of using that power or voice in a positive way? How can you use this newfound voice to establish boundaries that maintain your comfort level?

Disappointment

"For twenty years, I told myself that everything in my life would be better if I could lose the weight. Then I lost the weight, and the only thing that's different now is that I'm thinner."

"I thought that after I lost the weight people would no longer discriminate against me. Instead of discriminating against me for being fat, they now judge me for being pretty. I literally can't win for losing."

Losing weight *will* change your life. But those shed pounds will not make your job more interesting, your marriage more dynamic, your kids more responsible, or your mother-in-law less annoying.

It helps to have realistic expectations going into surgery, but you still may feel some disappointment. My most successful patients use the surgery as a catalyst, a first step in changing the other things in their lives that no longer bring them satisfaction. In fact, one of the greatest things for me about doing these surgeries is seeing the transformations they've been able to effect in the other parts of their lives as well.

Now that you've made this massive change in your life—a change you previously thought impossible—it's a good time to get in touch with the central kernel that is *you*.

Write your answers to these three questions on an index card:

- Who am I?

- What do I want?

- What is my purpose in this life?

In other words, how do you see yourself? What are your gifts? What do you feel you were put on this earth to do? What do you want your legacy to be? You've just gone through a period of intense self-reflection. How can you take what you've learned and use it to be of service to others, or to achieve goals and ambitions for yourself that you never allowed yourself to have before?

Check in with your answers to these three questions often; ideally carry them with you and repeat them to yourself every day. And don't be surprised when they change. These definitions of ourselves are constantly evolving—as they should.

Changing Relationships with People

"I'm included in a lot of things I wasn't included in before, and all I can think is, 'You would never be doing this if I still were fat.'"

"You learn real fast after surgery who your real friends are. I thought mine would be happy, but the reality is that I upset the balance."

People probably are treating you very differently now than they did when you were severely overweight. In truth, you're not the same person; you look and think a lot differently than you used to. But you feel like the same person much of the time, and it's natural to feel some anger, even if you're also flattered and enjoying the attention. You were just as funny and interesting and well-read and insightful before; you just were in a different body. How can the people you're meeting now be trusted? Would they have been willing to look beyond all that extra weight to find the person inside? You even may find, as one of my patients did, that people make fun of the overweight or obese in front of you, not knowing that you once walked in those shoes.

You need an outlet for these feelings. Going to an art class—one of Mary Jo's favorite recommendations—kills two birds with one stone. Creating something, whether it's a painting, a sculpture, or a macramé quilt, gives you a way to express your emotions creatively. And it gets you back into the mix, meeting people—new people, people who didn't know you "before"—so that you can get used to what that feels like.

Coping with Sadness or Depression

"Grief. I feel like I've gone through a bad breakup, or like someone close to me has died."

"I find that I am crying a lot. I hate myself for allowing the obesity to control so much of my life for so long. When will I ever allow myself to be happy?"

Many of my patients tell me that they grieve the loss of food much like they would grieve the loss of a dear friend. As you can imagine, this is painful. It's also a clear indication that food serves a purpose for you other than pure fuel.

In addition to grieving food, you may feel grief for the time you lost being overweight. You even may grieve for the person you were when you were obese. These are all natural reactions—this is a tough transition!—and a lot of weight-loss surgery patients experience them.

There's a medical reason for depression after surgery, too: Your hormonal balance is changing pretty rapidly. Remember, fat acts like an endocrine organ, releasing hormones. When your body-fat composition changes, your hormonal balance changes as well. If you've spent any time around a teen-ager, you know that hormonal changes set you up for changeable moods.

One exercise that we've found to be very helpful is to write a grief letter. Writing something down codifies it; it makes it more real than simply thinking it. And the act of writing a letter can be very powerful, which is why this is something we use again and again in support groups. You can write to whomever—or whatever—feels right to you: to an abuser, to a parent, to someone you've hurt. You can write to your presurgical self. We often recommend that people write a letter to their food, a "Dear John" let-ter to that unhealthy relationship.

It doesn't matter what you do with the letter once it's written. The point, as Mary Jo often says, is to "get it out of your head without eating it." Some patients burn their letters, others keep them, and some even share them with the special people in their lives. The letter isn't the point; the feelings are.

Unfortunately, if you have an addictive personality and are experienc-ing depression, it is possible that you may start looking for something to replace food. In the past, when you felt scared, depressed, lonely, disap-pointed, annoyed, or out of control, you ate, but now your pouch won't let you do that. It's important to find a healthy outlet for these feelings—as opposed to an unhealthy one, like spending too much money or drinking too much. Out of control bingeing, guilt feelings, and lying or justifying behaviors to family members and friends are all signs of possible addiction transfer. If you exhibit any of these behaviors or feelings, I strongly suggest that you find a counselor with experience in treating bariatric patients.

Sexual Unease

"I don't know what to do about the attention I get from men now. I was waiting for my friend at the bar the other night, and I was

*completely paralyzed by the looks I was getting; I felt like I was
naked. I ended up hiding in the ladies' room until she arrived."*

*"I never got to experience dating in my teens, twenties, or thir-
ties . . . I'm finding it hard not to act like a hormonal teenager,
saying yes to everyone who asks. I'm finally getting the attention
I never got before. I know this isn't healthy, but how do I stop? I
love how this new 'power' makes me feel."*

*"The thinner I get, the closer I get to the young girl who had all
those things happen to her. When I look in the mirror, my first
impulse is to protect her. Unfortunately, the only way I know
how to do that is by gaining weight."*

For some obese and formerly obese people, feeling like the object of
sexual attention causes a great deal of discomfort, and the increased attention that often comes with weight loss can be very unsettling for them.

Others, obese since childhood, tell us that they never learned to flirt or
date in high school the way their peers did. Now that they're being asked
out, they admit that they find it difficult to set boundaries for physical relationships, which may mean engaging in sexual behaviors with anyone
who finds them even remotely interesting. While this behavior may give
them a temporary feeling of euphoria—much like food did before—it is
destructive. It can also be dangerous, given the prevalence of sexually
transmitted diseases and the risk of unwanted pregnancy, to name just a
few hazards.

If you find yourself having difficulties setting boundaries in your physical relationships, I recommend that you meet with a counselor and ask
yourself some hard questions:

- Are you practicing safe sex every time? If not, why not?

- What feelings do you experience when you engage in these behaviors?

- Does having sex replace the way food made you feel before?

These are just some of the questions you will need to explore should
you find yourself acting out with excessive sexual behaviors.

Others find themselves squirming under the spotlight of sexual attention, literally paralyzed by any attention from the opposite sex.

For patients with a history of sexual abuse, this new sexual attention
can be extremely threatening and upsetting. If you're a survivor of sexual
abuse, it is imperative that you find someone to talk to about your experiences. Now that you're dismantling that hiding place, pound by pound, the
feelings are going to be very intense—and the compulsion to return to that
safe place by gaining weight will be very strong. You must recognize that
the abuse was not your fault and that you may have used excess weight as
a way of protecting yourself from further abuse.

Relationship Difficulties

*"My husband and I broke up about a year after my surgery. It's
terrible to say, but we weren't meant to be together; I married
him because I thought he was the best I could get."*

*"We're struggling a lot with jealousy right now. I'm getting a lot
of looks at bars and restaurants that I never used to get, and she's
not liking it very much. (I sort of am, though.)"*

*"I think my marriage is on the verge of breaking up. I think he
liked me being fat; it made him look like the one who had his life
together."*

I hate that this is true, but the fact is that bariatric patients do have a
higher incidence of relationship problems and divorce after surgery than
the general population. I'd be remiss not to address the issue.

One partner going through a massive change upsets the dynamic in any
partnership. As one of my patients said, "Once the dust settled, I realized
I didn't like what was still there." I take heart in the knowledge that many
of these relationships disintegrate because they just weren't right in the
first place, something that people figure out as they get healthier and more
confident in who they are.

If your marriage isn't strong, your weight loss may be the driver that
ends it. If your marriage is strong, your new commitment to better health
may bring you closer together. Whatever your circumstance, I highly rec-

ommend that you speak with your partner honestly about your concerns, fears, and feelings. Here are some recommendations from patients who have coped with these issues:

Do it together. You can't do it alone, and your spouse can be a very helpful advocate, particularly in large family settings where people may be less sensitive about your needs and less educated. But they can't help unless you include them, educate them, and allow them to participate in whatever you're going through. So bring them into the fold.

In my experience, it's a good thing for spouses to get on board, even if they're not obese. Who among us can't afford to eat a little more healthfully or to add a little more exercise into our lives? A lot of my patients institute a walk together after dinner; that's a perfect chance for you to spend some (healthy) time together.

One piece of advice a patient of mine had to offer: In the days and months after surgery, you're going to have to ask for a lot, so ask nicely. Even though you may be screaming inside, this is a time to use honey, not vinegar.

Talk about the changes. Your spouse may need support, too. Ask how he or she is experiencing your transformation. If you think it would help, ask your spouse to see a counselor with you or to see someone on their own.

Find new ways to be together. One patient told me that her husband was very reluctant to give up their big dinners, which had always been elaborate, gourmet, multicourse affairs. "I eat slowly and chew a million times, but, realistically, how long does it take to eat a chicken wing and a piece of broccoli?" she asked me at one follow-up appointment.

Of course, it wasn't the dinners he was missing, it was *her*—and the conversations they'd had over those many courses of food. So instead of picking up her novel after she was finished with her chicken wing, she made a conscious effort to stick around and talk—continuing the conversation they ordinarily would have had over the cheese course.

Process your frustration. Before surgery you didn't mind that he could eat anything he wanted and not gain a pound—you just went along and gained the weight. Now you realize just how unfair it is. And you may really resent the fact that he can go for the occasional scoop of ice cream on a hot summer's afternoon without dumping or worrying about what the scale will say tomorrow.

Those feelings have to be dealt with in a productive way—either in a support group, with a therapist, or in honest conversation with your spouse—so you don't end up taking it out on him in ways that hurt both of you.

Practice forgiveness. This may be the hardest one. Your spouse *is* going to mess up. He or she is going to forget and order a pizza, or buy a box of donuts at the supermarket, or make a joke about your rabbit food. As long as it's not part of a larger pattern of sabotage or emotional abuse, forgive and move on.

Impatience

"I'm frustrated by how long it's taking. I know I would have been ecstatic to see these numbers on the scale before surgery, but now I just can't wait to be thin and I'm not getting there fast enough!"

"It's easier than most of the diets I've been on, but it's still a diet."

I've said it before, and I'll say it again: Surgery is just a tool. You will have to modify your eating habits considerably and exercise often. And although the majority of people do lose quite a bit of weight very rapidly, it doesn't happen without a fair amount of effort. And it doesn't happen instantly.

One thing that does seem to help is looking at a pair of your old pants or photographs of yourself before surgery. In fact, I highly recommend that you take a photo at least once a month while you're losing. Keep a small photo album of these pictures, with notes of the date and your weight. Many of my patients hate the camera, but I tell them to grin and bear it; you'll cherish the photos after you reach your goal. And when you're feeling discouraged, like you haven't made any progress at all, these souvenirs of your old life allow you to see, in a very concrete way, how far you really have come.

Dysphoria

"I said, 'Excuse me'—and then walked right into the plate-glass window. For the first time in my life, I looked into something reflective and saw a normal person looking back at me."

"I was doing laundry and couldn't stop staring at a pair of my own jeans. It felt like I was going crazy. I finally asked my husband, 'Are you sure this is how small I am?'"

You've probably heard stories about bariatric patients who failed to recognize themselves when they saw themselves in a mirror or who accidentally bought clothes many sizes too big. These are all signs that there's a breakdown in reconciling who you used to be with who you are now.

That's natural—this is a big change for you to get used to (and maybe it will help you understand what everyone else in your life is going through as well). But the truth is, it's not good for us to feel disconnected from the bodies we're living in. You need to start seeing the person in the mirror as you and identifying their healthier habits as your own.

In order to bring the person you are in your mind's eye closer to the person who really exists in the world, try the following exercise:

Lie down on a piece of butcher block paper and have someone you trust intimately (a parent, a spouse, a friend) trace the outline of your body. Hang the result up on the wall. That's you! It's a true representation of the size you are now!

Mary Jo uses a number of different variations on this exercise. You can draw a heart over the part of your body that you feel was most negatively influenced by someone in your life. Or if you're struggling with body image, color the parts of your body you like the least with your least favorite color; the parts of your body that you feel neutral about with a beige; and the parts of your body that you love with your favorite color.

Struggles with Body Image

"Shopping for new clothes has been weird and stressful. I don't know what looks good on me now. And the weight's coming off so fast, I feel like I never have anything that fits."

"I was walking through the mall when I realized that I could go into any store and buy something off the rack, and it would fit. I stood there by myself—overwhelmed in the most glorious way—and cried tears of joy."

"I look great in clothes, but when I'm naked, I look like a melted candle. All this skin looks awful. Who is ever going to be attracted to this?!?"

As ecstatic as some of our patients are about finally getting to wear the latest fashions, many others find this task to be daunting and overwhelming. You may not have cared about how you dressed when you weighed more, but you will now, and you may need help in dressing "the new you."

Clothes aren't the only issue, either: "I weigh 400 pounds," one woman told Mary Jo before her surgery, "who's looking to see if I've plucked my eyebrows?" That's why the support groups where we invite a makeup expert, a hairstylist, or a clothing pro to come and speak are some of our most highly appreciated (by women, at least!).

It's important to invest time and energy in your appearance—and not just your body, but your hair, your skin, and your clothing and accessories. The way you present yourself to the world every day sends a message—what message do you send?

In support groups Mary Jo encourages everyone to buy a new outfit every six months. It doesn't have to be expensive, especially if you're still losing weight. But it does have to fit *who you are right now*. (Many support groups and online chat rooms have clothing swaps; this is an inexpensive way to find good-looking clothes that fit during your rapid weight-loss phase.)

Here are some other ways to reframe body image:

Think positive. When you think about your body, try not to focus on what it looks like but on what it can now do that it couldn't do before.

When your internal voice sends you a negative message, consciously replace it with something compassionate and affirming.

Don't focus on the numbers. If your eating and exercise habits are safely on track, you may find it helpful to take a short break from the scale and the tape measure. Ignoring them is unhealthy, but so is obsessing about them.

Turn off the culture. A blog recently printed the "before" and "after" photographs of a famous singer whose body and face had been digitally altered in a truly shocking way for her appearance on the cover of a woman's magazine. Her arms had been thinned, her crow's feet smoothed, her hair lightened, her lips plumped. If this woman—who is widely acknowledged to be one of the most beautiful in the country—doesn't pass muster, then who will?

If you find that you use images from our culture—the ones you see in magazines, on television, at the movies, and on billboards—as a launchpad for self-criticism, it may be time for a culture vacation.

Anxiety or Depression When Your Weight Loss Slows

"After losing seventy pounds in just under six months, I started to level off, and I got scared."

"After the rush wore off, I realized that all my old food hang-ups were still there—and that I was going to have to deal with them before the numbers on the scale started creeping up."

"I want my magic carpet back!"

After months of seeing really astonishing losses on the scale, your weight loss will slow—and eventually it will stop.

That's hard. It is very common for weight-loss surgery patients to experience some anxiety as weight loss begins to slow. Just as it does in marriage, reality sets in once the honeymoon is over. In this case, reality means slower weight loss—and, ultimately, it can mean that you stop short of your desired goal. Something else may be happening, too: For the first year, people probably were making a big fuss over you—over how much weight you were losing and how different you looked. Now the novelty has worn off, and "the new you" looks pretty much like you did last week. You may not be ready for all the hoopla to end.

Again, this is when your strong support network will play a vital role in your continued success. Listen to those who are further down the road and learn from their mistakes and victories. As one of my highly successful patients shared with me, "I realized that if I wanted to be successful, I needed to mimic the behaviors of successful people."

Instead of falling prey to depression or self-loathing messages in your head, push yourself a little harder and exercise more. Make sure your food choices are healthy ones, and revisit all of the basics. Remember to keep your follow-up visits, too. Staying connected to your surgeon and the practice most definitely will play an important role in your long-term success.

||||||||||||

I have one hope for all of my patients: that they can use the surgery to get healthy, and to learn to love who they are. If your BMI is less than 30 now, you went up against—and beat!—a deadly disease. Maybe you don't look like a model. But you've been through a great deal and you've accomplished a tremendous feat, and I hope you can see what I see: that the journey you've taken is cause for gratitude and celebration.

CHAPTER SIXTEEN

Excess Skin

And What to Do About It

"My husband calls me his shar-pei. It's not the prettiest thing in the world, but this skin is such a small price to pay for my health!"

"I felt less comfortable in my skinny body with all that extra skin than I did when I was fat."

Once you've lost your excess weight, you may find yourself coping with something else: excess skin. This is *very* common, especially in people who have lost over 100 pounds. Excess skin results from the skin stretching and losing its elasticity, so that when you lose the weight it doesn't snap back to fit your new, trimmer form.

Interestingly, it doesn't happen to everyone. Some people find themselves with just a little extra skin, while others are literally draped in excess tissue. The difference seems to be determined by a number of factors, including:

How overweight you got, and how much you've lost. Certainly the size you start out at does make a difference; someone who's lost 300 pounds probably is going to have more excess skin to deal with after they reach their goal weight than someone who's lost 75.

Your age. Young skin bounces back better and more quickly, I'm sorry to say. But even the young aren't immune to skin sag. In fact, if you've watched the show, you'll remember my patient Lauren who had a total body lift after losing close to 200 pounds, and she was in her late teens when she lost the weight.

Skin damage. People whose skin is damaged from too much sun worshipping are more likely to experience sag. Cigarette smoke also destroys collagen (which is why smokers tend to have more wrinkles), which can reduce elasticity.

Your genes. The real determining factor, in my opinion, is your genes. Some people get stretch marks during pregnancy; others don't. Some people lose weight and have tons of extra skin when they're done; others don't.

Unfortunately, the majority of these factors are out of your control. That's why all the folk remedies—drinking water, taking oil-based supplements—don't work.

WHAT ABOUT EXERCISE?

Probably the most prevalent old wives' tale about excess skin is that exercising while you're losing the weight and afterward will help to tighten the skin.

As much as I hate to take away a reason to exercise, it simply isn't true. Exercising won't tighten your skin; you simply can't do enough sit-ups to make enough muscle to fill it in. But you're not wrong if you think your excess skin looks better when you have a solid fitness program in place. Exercise does tighten the muscles that support the skin, which makes for a more toned appearance. And I personally believe that the improvement in the posture of someone who exercises regularly, and the grace and ease with which someone who is in shape moves, are big boons to one's appearance, no matter what your skin looks like.

Taking Care of Your Excess Skin

One of the very real problems associated with the excess skin that results from serious weight loss is the risk of skin infection or breakdown. Because this skin is already damaged, in a sense it has much less resilience and is at greater risk for infection. And the folds, which are hard to keep clean and dry, rub on each other, causing lacerations and ultimately infection. These infections can be painful, and they can lead to real complications; this is definitely something to stay in touch with your doctor about.

Ultimately, removing the skin entirely may be the best solution for you, and we'll talk about that in a minute. But following some basic care guidelines and using some products may help in the meantime.

Keep it clean! Shower often, particularly after exercise or when the weather is hot. Take the extra time in the shower to separate, lift, and clean each and every fold of skin. Use a surgical cleanser such as Hibiclens on the areas where you have trouble.

Keep it dry! Dry yourself very well after a shower, so that the skin inside all the folds is completely dry. Lots of bariatric patients air dry or use a hairdryer on the cold setting to dry the area completely before putting on clothes.

You'll also want to keep the susceptible areas as dry as you possibly can throughout the day. Obviously, you're going to sweat sometimes, especially if you work out or live in a warm climate, but do your best. Some of my patients like to use an absorbent medicated powder such as Gold Bond; a lot of them use plain old cornstarch, right out of the box. Others swear by products such as Moisture Barrier Salve from Kendall. An antichafing gel such as Monostat, applied to the areas where skin hangs over and becomes irritated, can also help.

Get in touch with your doctor. Call your PCP if your skin is bothering you. You shouldn't have to suffer, and prescription medications can be very helpful.

Keep a paper trail. If you have an infection, take pictures of the skin and make a note of your doctor's visits. Keep your prescription records and receipts for any over-the-counter medications your doctor recommends. As you'll see in a minute, this documentation is what an insurance company will need to see to approve you for reconstructive surgery.

Lift and separate. Compression garments—girdles and the like—can help. They will not only give you a cleaner line underneath your clothing, but they can also decrease friction and increase your functionality; a pair of compression shorts, for instance, can help you to walk without your thighs rubbing together. (For a list of suppliers, see page 207.)

Body Contouring

If you're someone who experiences difficulties as a result of excess skin, then you may want to consider a form of plastic surgery called body contouring. In 2003, more than 52,000 postbariatric plastic surgery procedures were performed, according to the American Society of Plastic Surgeons (ASPS). And those numbers are growing as bariatric surgery does.

Many people think of body contouring as a cosmetic procedure—and, unfortunately, that's the way most of the insurance companies think about it as well.

I don't agree.

Eliminating that excess skin after weight loss isn't about looking good, although it can be discouraging to go through the discomfort of surgery and the weight-loss process to be left with a body that's still marred by aprons of loose skin. But for me—and for most of my patients who end up getting the surgery—getting rid of that excess tissue is, first and foremost, a health issue.

I've seen patients who had to gather their belly skin up like a dress in order to walk. Even in less severe cases, excess skin poses a host of medical problems. It's uncomfortable and can make wearing clothes difficult—you may find yourself wearing two or three sizes above what you need to wear. Panels of redundant skin can make exercise difficult, which can lead to health problems and difficulty in maintaining your weight loss. And, as we've discussed, folds of skin rubbing against one another are subject to painful infections, rashes, and breakdown.

From a physician's point of view, addressing these issues surgically isn't cosmetic but *reconstructive*—meaning that it restores function. That said, you'll have to weigh the pros and cons for yourself.

Here's the short list:

The Cons

It's expensive. A body lift can cost anywhere between $30,000 and $50,000. Will your insurance pay for it? Probably not, because most of the insurance companies persist in seeing these as cosmetic procedures.

Scarring. The excess skin will be gone, but you'll always have scars. Plastic surgeons are, of course, adept at placing the scars where they're least likely to be seen—along the bikini line, for instance. And they will fade. But it's worth it to go to some plastic surgery Web sites to see what the scars look like a few years out to see if they're something you can live with.

It's painful, and there are risks. Plastic surgery is major surgery, and like all major surgeries, these procedures carry risks. And as relieved as you'll be to shed those excess folds, some patients are surprised to discover that the healing time is considerably longer and more painful than it was after their bypass.

The Pros

Surgery will resolve medical issues. As I said above, excess skin can present some very real medical issues, including discomfort, pain, and the risk of serious infection. Eliminate the excess skin, and you eliminate the problems.

It can boost self-esteem and help with remaining body issues. I've had patients who couldn't care less about the excess skin; I've had others who were bothered by it more than they were by being overweight. "I didn't go through so much and work so hard to end up with a body I feel ashamed of." For them the excess skin is an unhappy reminder of the obese person they used to be, and their transformation simply is not complete without the reconstruction.

I don't think that wanting to feel good about yourself is silly or shallow; in fact, quite the opposite: I believe that feeling good about yourself and the way you look is a fundamental part of being a healthy and happy person. If this is an issue for you, it will weigh heavily in the pro column.

Finding a Surgeon

If you decide to pursue plastic surgery, I'd suggest that you look for a plastic surgeon with experience in these kinds of procedures—in other words, someone who has done a number of body contouring procedures on people who have excess skin as a result of massive weight loss. Doing a full body lift on a 125-pound woman who has lost 300 pounds is different than doing a tummy tuck on a 125-pound woman who lost some muscle tone after a cesarean, so you'll want to make sure that your surgeon has lots of experience with postbariatric surgeries.

Your weight-loss surgeon almost certainly has someone that he or she works with on a regular basis. If not, the American Society of Plastic Surgeons has a searchable database on their Web site, PlasticSurgery.org, as does the bariatric support Web site, ObesityHelp.com.

Talking to Your Plastic Surgeon. Plastic surgeons generally have portfolios of before and after photographs, which can be very instructive. The questions you may want to ask your plastic surgeon at your consultation may include:

Where will the surgery be performed?
What are the risks of the procedure?
How long is the recovery period? How long before you can go back to work/drive a car?
What can I do—now, and after surgery—to ensure that I get the best results possible?

One answer we've gotten is unanimous: Keep your protein up! Protein levels directly affect the quality of the skin and its ability to heal. This is yet another reason to make sure your nutrition is flawless. And, of course, don't smoke.

Convincing Your Insurance Company

This is, in all likelihood, going to be a harder battle than the one you waged to get your bariatric surgery. Your best weapon is to do your homework and be completely, meticulously prepared.

Read your policy. Elective plastic surgery is hardly ever covered. Medically necessary reconstructive surgery sometimes is. Figure out what you'll need to do to prove that your surgery is medically necessary. Check the online support groups; you'll often find that someone on a board has already danced with your insurance company and can tell you specifically what helped or hurt their case.

Document EVERYTHING! If you want to have your case considered seriously, documentation is king.

Important! Don't wait until you reach your goal weight to begin documentation.

The file you submit should contain:

- A letter from you detailing why you want the skin removed. Stay focused on what the insurance company cares about. They don't, I'm sorry to say, care if you feel bad on the beach or if you have a hard time fitting into clothes. They're worried about the stuff they're probably going to have to pay for down the line—such as recurring infections.

- Letters from your doctors: your PCP, surgeon, dermatologist, chiropractor, OB/GYN, plastic surgeon—anyone who can vouch for the medical necessity of this surgery. If the skin or back pain prevents you from exercising, for instance, you'll want to include medical letters saying so.

- A detailed description of your skin-care regimen; what you do to prevent skin breakdown and what you do when you have an infection, for example. Include labels and receipts of your prescriptions for related antibiotics and skin creams.

- Photographs of hanging skin. A picture is worth a thousand words. Some patients take pictures every few months as they lose the weight, with a notation of the date and the amount of weight lost.

- Photographs of open wounds, rashes, and sites of irritation.

As always, make copies and send the copies—keep your originals! And if your surgeon is preparing the letter for the insurance company, ask to read it before it goes out. Nobody knows your issues as well as you do.

Again, even with these measures, the rate of approval for these surgeries is absolutely abysmal. You can, of course, talk to your surgeon about a payment plan; many of them will accommodate you or can direct you to a company that specializes in medical loans.

HOW LONG SHOULD I WAIT BEFORE CONSIDERING RECONSTRUCTIVE SURGERY?

You'll want to wait until you've reached your goal weight, and stayed there for a while. Recommendations vary, anywhere from a year to two years. Make sure you're done losing! You wouldn't want to have the surgery and then lose more weight, causing more excess skin.

Which Surgery Is Right for You?

There are a number of common body contouring surgeries after weight loss. I turned to a surgeon at Methodist Hospital in Houston (and a regular on *Big Medicine*), Dr. Norman Rappaport, to walk us through some of them:

Breast surgery. Breast tissue is mostly fat, so this is one of the areas that tends to sag when great amounts of weight are lost. Surgery is available to raise the remaining breast tissue, a procedure called a breast lift, or mastopexy. Women sometimes opt for implants, or augmentation, at the same time; as the fat disappears, so, often, do the breasts.

Men who have lost a great deal of weight may also find themselves with gynecomastia, or excess breast tissue. This can be removed and the skin lifted, bringing the chest back to a more masculine profile. In addition, the nipples sometimes are very stretched out; they can be reduced to give them a more normal appearance.

Brachioplasty. Weight-loss surgery veterans sometimes call the excess skin that's left on their upper arms their batwings. These panels of excess skin can be removed so that the skin more closely follows the shape of the arm. This is a very common surgery, and a successful one, although it does leave scars on the inside of your arms that can be seen if you're wearing something sleeveless.

Thighplasty. Excess skin on the inside of the thigh can make walking and exercise very difficult. That skin can be removed, and what remains can be lifted.

Abdominoplasty. Also known as a tummy tuck. In this surgery, the excess skin is removed, the abdominal muscles are tightened, and (if possible) the belly button is repositioned. There are many variations on this theme. There is the panniculectomy, which is simply an amputation of the excess skin. This is simple, has lower complication rates, and is less painful than the other types. It is also less likely to give you the cosmetic result you're looking for, but if all you care about is eliminating that belly overhang so that skin care is easier, this is a great procedure.

If you really want to tighten up your whole abdomen, a true abdominoplasty with belly tightening (called "undermining") is the procedure of choice. During this procedure, excess skin is removed and the remaining skin is lifted up off the abdomen and pulled down tight. The muscles are also tightened. This will leave you with a very flat abdomen and actually will remove some scars and stretch marks. The scars from the surgery are typically made in the bikini line, so eventually you'll be able to look great in one. This is a much more involved surgery with greater risks of infection and pain.

Neck- or face-lift. The skin of the face and neck are not immune to sag after weight loss. Sometimes it's very dramatic, and patients opt to have this skin lifted.

Total body lift. This is really a combination of procedures: a tummy tuck, a thigh lift, and a bottom lift. It is also known as a belt lipectomy, and it is very effective at reshaping the torso and lower body. This is one of the most common procedures my patients have done. Because it means lifting the back as well as the front, some surgeons will do this procedure as two separate surgeries at two different times.

An added bonus: You'll also lose weight! On *Big Medicine*, Dr. Jeffrey Friedman, the head of plastic surgery at Methodist Hospital, removed what turned out to be about twenty-five pounds of loose skin from one of my patients, Kim. Dr. Rappaport removed sixty pounds from another patient, Allan.

Many patients opt to get a number of these surgeries done at the same time. Talk to your surgeon about what they recommend: If there are complications, they may not be able to keep you under anesthesia for long enough to do multiple procedures, and having a number of different areas done extends your recovery time. Of course, you'll also get it over with, and you won't have to take separate chunks of time off work.

DONATE WHAT YOU DON'T NEED!

The Musculoskeletal Transplant Foundation (MTF) has a Living Skin donation program, which means that the excess skin that's removed during your plastic surgery can be donated to help burn victims and other people who need tissue. Ask your surgeon about participating, or visit the Musculoskeletal Transplant Foundation Web site, MTF.org.

After Your Surgery

Make sure you've got someone to take care of you after surgery; by all accounts, these procedures tend to have more painful recoveries than weight-loss surgery, and you'll quite likely have limited mobility for a while afterward.

In the weeks following surgery, you'll be pretty bruised and swollen. Don't panic! You won't be able to see results immediately after the surgery, although what's been accomplished should still be pretty apparent. Your surgeon will recommend compression garments (patients often find that wearing a light T-shirt, like a man's sleeveless tank-top-style undershirt underneath these garments prevents chafing and helps the skin to breathe). You may feel some "zapping" electrical sensations for a while as the nerves regenerate, and the swelling and tenderness around the incision may last for a few months.

CHAPTER SEVENTEEN

Negotiating Pitfalls

"I hadn't had a piece of candy in a year. But there was something about the way the chocolate in my son's Easter basket smelled that sent me completely around the bend."

"It was scary when my dad got really sick; I was stressed and too busy, and I saw how easy it would be to fall into old patterns."

All WLS patients will find themselves facing down temptation at some point in their journey. In this chapter we'll go through some of the common pitfalls that lie in wait for WLS patients—and we'll give you some strategies to make sure they don't trip you up.

Before we begin, I'd like to point out some common threads I've noticed in people's ability to successfully negotiate pitfalls.

1) **Self-awareness:** You have to know where temptation lies *for you*. One of my patients told me that she's never been tempted by food at a cocktail party: "As long as I have a glass of water with lime in one hand, there's enough to distract me." But others know that the waiters might as well have hand grenades on those little trays. Know thyself—and act accordingly.

2) **Problem solving:** Plan ahead. It does require a little forethought to make sure that you've got enough time to pack yourself a healthy lunch in the morning—but without that healthy lunch, you're more likely to order in from the greasy Chinese place. Pack your containers the night before or set the alarm fifteen minutes early so you can pack them before you leave. Spotting the problems ahead of time allows you to figure out how you're going to solve them.

3) **Support:** It's not accidental that lots of these traps involve other people. The brunt of educating the other people in your life about weight-loss surgery is going to fall to you. Only when your coworkers understand that you're hypersensitive to alcohol and sugar will they stop pushing that happy hour margarita on you. And, even armed with that knowledge, there's no guarantee that they've got your best interests in mind. Surround yourself with people who are supportive, and give them the information they need to help so that you have somewhere to turn to when the going gets tough—as it will sometimes.

Potential Pitfall #1:
The Not-So-Supportive Support System

"I think you're getting too thin; you don't look healthy."

"These used to be your favorite; I spent all day making them just for you. Have one, for me."

"You lost a lot of weight, but it's not like you really did anything."

"That has a lot of mayonnaise in it; are you sure you should be eating that?"

Steam coming out of your ears yet? These are all statements that my patients have heard over the years from friends and family—and there are plenty more where those came from.

Hopefully the majority of the people in your life will be supportive of your new lifestyle. But, unfortunately, not everybody will be. Here are some tactics you can use to make sure your relationships don't slow your progress rather than promote it.

Education. Your first line of defense is clear, open communication. Let's face it: You've immersed yourself in this new WLS world, but your friends and family haven't, and they may not realize that their comments sound like criticisms or that their actions feel like sabotage. So tell them, in as clear and kind a way as possible, with statements like: "It's really hard for me to stay with my program when I know there's ice cream in the freezer. Could I ask you instead to get a cone at the ice-cream store when I'm not with you?"

If the people in your life seem open to learning more about what you're going through and how they can help, you could even suggest that they read something (this book, for instance) or come to a support group with you.

And it's good to remember that even the most supportive and well-meaning friend or family member is going to do the wrong thing sometimes.

Avoid the situation. If you feel like your portion sizes and food choices are under a microscope when you go out to dinner with friends, suggest a movie instead. And if the topic of conversation rolls around to dieting or food in an unproductive way, change the subject. The novelty of your surgery and weight loss will wear off eventually; it just may take a little time.

Blame your doctor! We don't mind being the bad guys. When my wife was pregnant, people periodically would come up to her and offer unsolicited advice. (For some reason, the more likely someone is to butt in, the less they always seem to know.) She found that it was very effective to smile sweetly and tell people that she was doing whatever she was doing with the full knowledge and approval of her OB/GYN.

Similarly, if someone is giving my patients a hard time, I tell them to shut the conversation down by invoking doctor's orders with a response like: "My nutritionist/dietician/surgeon was very specific about portion sizes; I'm following her instructions to the letter." You know what you need to do.

Don't be pushed. No matter how long your mother slaved over a hot stove to make those cookies, you're not supposed to eat them. If she knows that and made them anyway, then there's something else going on.

The most productive thing to do would be to use the incident as the spark for a larger conversation. But even if you don't feel up to that, have the strength of your convictions, and just say no.

You don't have to be rude, just firm. Even if you feel silly doing it, it may help to role-play some polite but definite responses in advance, like "Thank you so much for thinking of me! I'm so sorry that eating those will make me ill" or "My health won't permit me to have any, but I'll enjoy watching you have some!"

As awkward as it might be to reject these offerings in the moment, you'll feel much better for standing up for yourself than you will if you cave—and you won't have established a dangerous precedent.

Walk away. Like it or not, there are going to be people who feel threatened by your new success, and they may—consciously or unconsciously—set you up to fail.

You'll know who they are. Instead of complimenting you on how much healthier you look, they'll find something to disparage. Instead of feeling supported in your choices, you'll feel like you're constantly under attack. Your time with these people will exhaust and deplete you, and you may find that you suddenly feel bad about yourself or doubtful about your path when you're with them.

If none of the above strategies defuse the situation, you may end up phasing the friendship out of your life. This probably is a pretty scary thing to hear, but I can say with some confidence that I don't know a single person who, overall, is less happy with their social life or friendships after surgery than they were when they were obese.

Potential Pitfall #2:
Plateaus

"You're doing everything right, and it's like the scale is stuck. It's okay for a couple of days, and then you start thinking, if this isn't working, then what am I doing it for?"

The truth is that you're going to hit a plateau, a time when your weight loss slows down or even stops for a period of time before you've reached your goal weight. It *will* happen—it does to almost everyone. And while it can be very alarming for someone who has gotten used to the pounds flying off, it is completely natural for the rate at which you lose to slow down, and even to stop for a bit.

Now, there are some very specific, prescriptive things you can do to jolt your body out of this plateau, and we'll get to those in a minute. But in my experience, the real danger here is psychological. In and of itself, a slowdown or plateau is not a pitfall—but it can turn into one if you're not careful to approach it the right way.

You see, it's dangerously easy, particularly for people who have struggled with their weight for a long time, to give in to the feeling of failure. You're probably the veteran of a thousand diets, none of which helped you to achieve permanent weight loss. So the feeling that you're failing now is going to be very familiar. But just because it's familiar doesn't mean it's good for you, so don't give in! Failure is a self-fulfilling prophecy.

Instead:

Get some perspective on what's really happening. You are genetically predisposed to obesity, which means that when you start losing weight quickly, your body is going to rebel. Your body translates weight loss into "I'm starving!" which is why your metabolic rate is slowing.

Remind yourself of what's different this time. This time you're not battling against your body; instead, you have a tool to help you make the right choices.

Remind yourself, as often as you need to:

**You are battling a disease,
and you are winning.**

Stay positive! Don't forget that how you think is an enormous component in your success. Some of my patients meditate for fifteen minutes every morning on the idea that they are successful and will be successful. Some of them leave themselves Post-it notes on the refrigerator, the bathroom mirror, and their computer screen that say "You are a success." Let it be the first thing you say to yourself in the morning and the last thing you say to yourself at night.

Be patient. As long as you're not overeating or making poor choices, you're going to get off this hump. Your body will settle into this new weight, and you'll be ready to lose again; it just takes a little time. In fact, a very common losing pattern is a dip in one's weight, followed by a plateau, followed by another dip, and then another plateau. Let your body get comfortable while you keep doing what you're supposed to do, and the pounds will start coming off again.

Now that your mind's in order, let's get down to the nitty-gritty. Something is happening—it's time to find out what it is.

Is there really a problem? This is the first question to ask yourself. Sometimes the numbers of the scale don't budge—even though you're dropping sizes. Take your measurements (or just pay attention to the way your clothes fit). Maybe this isn't a plateau after all, just a time when you're losing inches and not pounds.

This is fairly common when people start to get fitter; after all, muscle weighs more than fat does. If you're doing everything right and you look good, then there's nothing to worry about; the scale will catch up with your waistband eventually.

Is there a medical reason for your slowdown? Have you been sick or have you added a medication? Women may notice that their weight loss slows or stalls in the week leading up to their menstrual period.

Has something else changed in your life? Life changes can dramatically influence our diet and habits, sometimes without us realizing it. Maybe the kids are out of school for the summer, so you've been finding it hard to get to the gym every day. Or you're traveling a lot for work and struggling to make good choices from a room service menu. Are you very busy? That's not an excuse to eat more than you normally would or to get off your exercise schedule; eating properly and exercising will help, not hurt. Take stock of the situation and make adjustments as necessary.

Check your stress level, too. A study on rats showed that when they were under chronic stress, they secreted more stress hormones, specifically one called cortisol, which led to a greater distribution of fat in their belly. Cortisol has the same effect in humans.

Watch out for calorie creep. The best way to be entirely sure about what you're eating is to do your food preparation at home. Tuna salad made with a reasonable amount of low-fat mayonnaise and mixed with healthy vegetables might look and taste pretty similar to the one you get from the local deli, but the difference might be as great as a few hundred calories and 20 grams of fat.

Increase your water intake. Make sure you're drinking enough water. It's easy to mistake the feeling of being thirsty for hunger, and drinking enough between meals—not with them—will also make you feel full.

Green tea has metabolism-boosting properties (100 percent brewed green tea, not the green-tea-flavored drinks you can buy, which are only slightly better than soda). Brew a pot every day, and drink it, adding noncaloric sweeteners if you need them. It might give your metabolism the kickstart it needs.

Get back to basics. Literally—go back to page 142, photocopy that page, and put it where you can see it. If it's been a while since your surgery, your portion sizes may have crept up; it's time to dust off the scale and use your measuring cups again. Are you grazing without realizing it? Before you pop what's left of your kid's grilled cheese into your mouth as you clean up the lunch dishes, think seriously about whether you want to put it down in your food journal. Are you drinking water with some meals? Beware this pitfall. Plan your meals carefully, and make sure you don't leave the house without a healthy snack. In other words, do what you did at the very beginning.

Are you cheating? Make sure you're not sabotaging yourself. In truth, you can cheat a little bit without paying the price—but that's a self-defeating behavior. You end up saying, "See? I had potato chips with my lunch yesterday, and I didn't gain any weight!" Of course, if you make that a regular occurrence, you are going to see an upward trend in your weight. Don't "just one bite" yourself back to obesity.

Exercise. This is the big one. *Nothing* increases your metabolism and gets the scale moving again like getting moving.

Exercise is *the* plateau-buster.

Unfortunately, exercise is a perfect example of the law of diminishing returns. If your body has gotten used to one intensity level, you're going to stop seeing results. In order to keep seeing progress, you're going to have to ramp it up.

You have to *really* exercise. When you were very obese, just walking might have been enough—but, now that you're more fit, it probably isn't. Strength training builds muscle, which increases your metabolic rate. Get your heart rate up into the desired zone—and keep it there for half an hour or more.

Consider adding another session. If you're working out three times a week, adding a fourth session at the gym—or even just a long, medium-paced walk on one of your off days—may do the trick.

Try interval training. Interval training is alternating periods of more intense cardiovascular work with less intense periods. For instance, if you walk on the treadmill, try adding short periods of very rapid walking or jogging. Do twenty jumping jacks as you're moving from one weight training exercise to the next. It's not a lot of added effort, but it keeps your heart rate up and helps you to burn more calories.

Increase your time. If you usually get off the treadmill after half an hour, see if you can add a few minutes every session until you get to forty-five minutes or an hour.

Change it up. As you might remember from Chapter 14, the body not only gets used to certain intensity levels but to certain types of exercise as well. If you walk on the treadmill, try the bike instead. Try yoga or Pilates if you've never done them before.

Get help. Personal trainers are expensive, but I recommend that my patients splurge on a few sessions a couple of times a year if possible—particularly if they're struggling to get off a plateau. If that's simply out of the question for you, consider taking a group class at the gym or making very specific fitness goals for you to achieve.

Potential Pitfall:
Eating in Restaurants

"Our favorite restaurant is the hardest part for me. I want a beer, and what I used to order!"

I prefer that my patients limit dining out to two times a week; in fact, we'd all be a lot healthier if we did more cooking at home.

That said, eating in restaurants is a fact of life—and today Americans eat out more than they ever have before. And it can be hard! Even people who don't struggle with obesity have a hard time eating moderately in restaurants. There's a festivity in the air that naturally gives way to an "anything goes" mentality. Portion sizes are enormous—often three to five times a normal serving size, which means enough for six to ten meals for someone after WLS. And if you've ever eaten in a restaurant with an open kitchen, you know that everything tastes so good because *fat* tastes good—an ingredient that professional kitchens don't stint on! But with a little planning and some tricks, you can enjoy eating out without going off plan.

Get a headstart. Many restaurants feature their menus on their Web sites. Sometimes they even include nutritional information! Take time at home to peruse the offerings, and make a decision about what you're going to eat before you get there. It's much easier to make healthy decisions when there's no time pressure or temptation of the "oh, *that* sounds good" variety.

Send the bread back. At most restaurants, you're presented with two or three meals worth of calories—and before you've even ordered! Don't let the bread basket (or the chip basket in a Mexican restaurant) even hit the table. Just tell the waiter you won't be needing it, thank you very much.

Order healthfully. Don't hesitate to ask questions of your server; you may even want to explain that you've had bariatric surgery and that extra fat or sugar can make you sick. Menu words to avoid include: au gratin, escalope, cheese sauce, creamed, parmesan, hashed, marinated in oil, served in its own gravy, and pot pie.

Steamed and boiled vegetables are a better choice than sautéed; ask for them plain, without butter or oil. Similarly, sautéed, fried, and pan-fried meats and fish will come with more fat than you want or need; choose broiled or baked options instead. Choose lean proteins, and substitute unhealthy sides—french fries, mashed potatoes, and so on—with a green salad or some steamed vegetables.

Salad dressings and sauces often provide more calories than the stuff they go on, so ask for them on the side and dip your fork in them before eating, instead of pouring them over.

Control portion sizes. One of the biggest issues in restaurants is portion control. Restaurants serve too much food—and, as you know, the more you have in front of you, the more you're going to eat.

Order an appetizer; appetizers often are the perfect portion size for someone after surgery. Sometimes they're even too big! Or ask if you can have a child-size portion. In my practice, we print a card for our patients that they can laminate and carry in their wallet:

> **The bearer of this card has had bariatric**
> **weight-loss surgery.**
> **Please allow them to order a child-size or**
> **senior portion, or to split an adult-size portion**
> **without a share charge.**

Ask your surgeon's office if they can provide you with something similar.

If that doesn't work, ask the waiter for a to-go container *with* your food—not afterward. As soon as the food arrives, move everything over and above a healthy portion into the to-go container. You may discover that you're taking home enough for two or three meals!

Slow down. Armed with a big plate and a big fork, and engrossed in a heated conversation about the movie star meltdown du jour, you may not notice that you've eaten too much—or too quickly—until you're running to the bathroom to get rid of those extra bites.

Potential Pitfall #3:
The Holidays

"There is junk EVERYWHERE during the holidays. You buy a dress, there are snowball chocolates in a bowl at the checkout counter. There are candy canes at the dry cleaner and Christmas cookies at the office. It's crazy how many temptations you find yourself confronting, just in the normal course of the day. Did I just not notice before I got banded? Or maybe I just didn't notice what I was putting in my mouth."

It's said that Americans gain about ten pounds between October and January. Between the Halloween candy, the Thanksgiving turkey, honey cake on Rosh Hashanah, and the Sugar Plum Fairy, these months are minefields for someone who's trying to comply with a healthy diet. Many people cope with the cold and shortened days with comfort food and carbs—who will know, under those all those layers and bulky coats?

As special as the holidays are, and as intrinsically linked as they are to special foods for many people, they're not a reason to get off your program. You have a lot to celebrate; just remember your basics, and do it healthfully.

Celebrate the seasons with events that aren't food-related. Take your family to select a Christmas tree or go ice-skating; play football on the lawn instead of watching the halftime show with beer and wings during the big game. Make sure there's lots of stuff to do at the barbecue— badminton, slip and slide, croquet—besides eating.

Don't use being busy as an excuse. Yes, your schedule is likely crowded: There are parties to plan, pageants to attend, and presents to buy, and not enough time to do it all. But all this running around *isn't* an excuse for you not to fit in your fitness program, to eat more than you would normally, or to choose foods that aren't healthy. If you're going to be out all day shopping or running errands, pack healthy snacks, and have a small meal or a protein shake before you leave.

Out of sight, out of mind. Wherever you can, eliminate temptations by removing them from sight. If your client sends a giant tub of caramel popcorn every year at the holidays, send a thank-you note, and then get it out of the break room. Ask your colleagues to take what they want, and then throw the rest out. One mom I know lets her kids eat whatever they want on Halloween night but then swaps the remainders for a coveted video game or DVD, while the candy goes in the trash. "No matter what I spend, it's worth it not to have that junk in the house."

Go back to your support group. Find out how others are coping with the challenges of the season; share your own struggles—and successes. One great way to get through the holidays is to throw a party at your support group. Ask everyone to bring something compliant and have a great time!

Give them up! If holidays are a really bad time for you, consider giving them up—for a little while. A patient of mine whose operation was at the end of the summer decided not to attend Thanksgiving dinner the first year. "I knew I couldn't handle all that food on the table; I just knew I'd end up dumping and sick." So, with the blessings of her family, she skipped the dinner altogether.

She did turn up afterward for her family's traditional walk around the neighborhood, and she did take home a small packet of turkey leftovers so she wouldn't feel completely deprived. I think she'll probably be established enough in her habits to be fine next year. But I also think she was right to take herself out of the line of temptation when she knew she wouldn't be able to handle it.

BRIBE YOURSELF!

I know that a number of my patients bribe themselves for passing up a poor food choice that they're finding particularly tempting. "I tell myself that I'll make time for a manicure the next day," one of my patients told me. Another, with an expensive model train hobby, banks a dollar in a jar toward a new train for every snack cake he doesn't eat.

Be cautious with this strategy; we're not looking for you to get into financial trouble or to trade a food addiction for a shopping addiction. But if the idea of a little something special will steer you away from an unhealthy choice, then treat yourself—with something you can't eat.

Potential Pitfall #4:
Parties

"I spend a lot of time at trade shows for work, and there's always a cocktail party with wine and lots of little things on toothpicks. I love those guys. But you have to be careful not to eat a whole day's calories while you're shooting the breeze."

Parties can be difficult for the same reasons that the holidays and restaurants are hard. Temptations abound, and spirits run high—and there are lots of distractions, so it can be hard to really pay attention to the quality and the quantity of the food you're eating.

Eat a little something before. You don't want to be starving when you arrive; your hunger will make it hard to choose wisely. If you're not ravenous, you'll be able to stand back, relax, and then choose foods that fit with your program. Not all traditional party snacks are unhealthy; you just have to make sure you're concentrating on the crudités, not on the dip.

Don't skip meals, hoarding your daily calories for a big splurge—the "starve and stuff" cycle is not only unpleasant; it's a disaster waiting to happen.

Bring something you know you'll be able to eat. If you know there's going to be a groaning buffet table, offer to bring your own dish so you know there definitely will be something delicious there for you. It also ensures that there's something for you to eat that you know won't make you sick. Parties aren't a good time to try a lot of new foods, even healthy ones; you don't want to have to go home early with an upset stomach.

Pay attention. The same rules apply at parties as in everyday life: protein first, no drinking while eating, and small portions. Once you've made your healthy choices, move away from the food; don't stand and snack straight from the buffet table, or you may end up eating quite a bit more than you intended to. Band patients often tell me that they got caught up in party conversation and failed to chew something as well as they should have—nothing puts a stop to that pleasant chat like a dash to the bathroom! Enjoy yourself, but concentrate on what you're doing.

Avoid the bar. I ask my bypass patients in particular to avoid alcohol for the first year after surgery, and many of them find that they don't go back afterward because the change in the way they metabolize alcohol means that it takes very little for them to become intoxicated.

Alcohol is loaded with nonnutritive calories, and being even a little bit tipsy makes it hard to make good choices. If you are drinking again, consider choosing not to in a high-temptation situation like a party.

SLIP-UP, OR SLIPPERY SLOPE?

If you do overeat on a special occasion or on just a regular old day, keep it in perspective. It's not the end of the world; what really matters is what you do on a daily basis. Don't punish yourself, either—just eat sensibly again, starting as soon as you possibly can.

The difference between success and failure is the ability to dust yourself off and get back on the horse.

What you really want to avoid is the "Well, the day is shot—I might as well eat whatever I want to and start over tomorrow" mentality. That's the slippery slope. Correct the mistake by eating healthfully at your very next meal.

Potential Pitfall #5
I'm Cured!

"I'm an obese person in a thin person's body, and I think that's the way it's always going to be."

A trim friend tells you she can't remember the last time she went to the gym; a movie star on a talk show brags about how much red meat she eats; your boyfriend polishes off a giant plate of nachos and doesn't have an extra pound of body fat. And you start to think, "Hey, if they can do it, maybe I can, too. . . ."

It's very tempting, especially after you've lost a lot of weight, to think that you've been permanently cured of your obesity. You don't see your former self when you look in the mirror—maybe she really is gone forever!

Well, here's the truth, and it's something you're going to want to remember, even if it's not what you want to hear: You are not one of those people who can eat anything you want and still maintain a healthy weight. You are not someone who can slack off for a few months at the gym and stay in great shape. Just as you will have to take supplements for the rest of your life in order to stay healthy, *you will have to watch what you eat and keep your activity level high for the rest of your life in order to maintain your new weight.*

Feel free to be as mad as you want about the injustice of this—you can shake your fist at the sky and curse your genes all day long if you want to. Just don't ignore the reality, even if it's painful. Look back at photographs taken before you lost the weight. Remember the medications you had to take, the aches and pains you contended with every day, the embarrassment and the stares. Talk to other WLS patients—every single one of them will know exactly what you're going through!

Ultimately I know you'll decide that—as unfair as it might be—exercising daily and sticking to small portions of healthy foods is the way you want to live.

Conclusion

||||||||||||||||||||||||||||||||||||||||||||||||||||||||||||||

"I felt and acted like an old person. Now I don't. It's as simple as that."

In 2006, the American Society for Metabolic and Bariatric Surgery reported that an estimated 177,600 people in the United States have had bariatric surgery. That's a pretty impressive number.

But as impressive as that number may be, it pales in comparison with the number of people suffering from obesity in this country. The ASMBS, in fact, puts that at about 1 percent, if you accept that 15 million people in this country qualify as morbidly obese.

**Less than 2 percent of those who meet the criteria
for surgery actually have surgery.**

Now trust me: I'm not hunting for patients—it's all I can do to keep my waiting room from looking like Grand Central Station. But as a doctor, those numbers trouble me.

Every day in my office I see the wages of untreated obesity. This, after all, is not just a disease in its own right but one that gives way to a cascade of twenty or more other, often life-threatening, diseases. I have seen the physical toll obesity takes on the people who live with it: the out-of-control type 2 diabetes, asthma, heart disease, high blood pressure, arthritis, and cancer. I see the emotional toll, too. And I have been lucky enough to see how people can transform their lives when their joints no longer hurt, their infertility is resolved, and the snickering and hurtful comments stop.

So the idea that *less than 2 percent* of the people suffering from this disease are getting the help they need is unacceptable to me. Doctors take an oath to help people—and yet, as I discussed at the beginning of this book, it is common medical practice to send obese people out of their offices with advice—"eat less and exercise"—that has been scientifically proven not to help them.

Too few people are getting the help they need.

If you're contemplating surgery, I hope that what you have found in this book gives you a realistic idea of how much will be required of you. It was never my intention to write a book glibly implying that the pounds will drop off without effort, and that thinner thighs and toned arms are just around the corner. There are enough of those books on the market already, and I'd have to answer every day to my patients, who know the truth. Surgery is not a cure-all but a tool. In order for it to be a successful intervention over the long term, a tremendous amount of education and sheer effort are required on the part of the patient.

And you can't do it alone. Succeeding after surgery will require you to have a rich, multilayered support system. That support will come from the professionals you bring into your life, from family and friends who are glad and grateful to assist you on this path to a healthier life, and from the rich, vibrant, opinionated community of WLS patients out there. After surgery, this support system will be a necessity; I think you will come to find, as many of my patients have, that it is also a collateral benefit.

Weight-loss surgery may not be an easy road, but it is one that works. These procedures can offer a beacon of hope after a lifetime of diet failures. And their success at resolving some of the most insidious co-morbidities associated with obesity—diseases including heart disease, arthritis, and especially diabetes—cannot be overlooked. I believe that these surgeries can mean the gift of life to the 15 million obese people in this country. And from the thousands of people I've treated, I know just what that gift can mean.

Appendix A

Body Mass Indexes

BMI	19	20	21	22	23	24	25	26	27	28	29	30	31	32	33	34	35
Height (inches)	Body Weight (pounds)																
58	91	96	100	105	110	115	119	124	129	134	138	143	148	153	158	162	167
59	94	99	104	109	114	119	124	128	133	138	143	148	153	158	163	168	173
60	97	102	107	112	118	123	128	133	138	143	148	153	158	163	168	174	179
61	100	106	111	116	122	127	132	137	143	148	153	158	164	169	174	180	185
62	104	109	115	120	126	131	136	142	147	153	158	164	169	175	180	186	191
63	107	113	118	124	130	135	141	146	152	158	163	169	175	180	186	191	197
64	110	116	122	128	134	140	145	151	157	163	169	174	180	186	192	197	204
65	114	120	126	132	138	144	150	156	162	168	174	180	186	192	198	204	210
66	118	124	130	136	142	148	155	161	167	173	179	186	192	198	204	210	216
67	121	127	134	140	146	153	159	166	172	178	185	191	198	204	211	217	223
68	125	131	138	144	151	158	164	171	177	184	190	197	203	210	216	223	230
69	128	135	142	149	155	162	169	176	182	189	196	203	209	216	223	230	236
70	132	139	146	153	160	167	174	181	188	195	202	209	216	222	229	236	243
71	136	143	150	157	165	172	179	186	193	200	208	215	222	229	236	243	250
72	140	147	154	162	169	177	184	191	199	206	213	221	228	235	242	250	258
73	144	151	159	166	174	182	189	197	204	212	219	227	235	242	250	257	265
74	148	155	163	171	179	186	194	202	210	218	225	233	241	249	256	264	272
75	152	160	168	176	184	192	200	208	216	224	232	240	248	256	264	272	279
76	156	164	172	180	189	197	205	213	221	230	238	246	254	263	271	279	287

BMI	36	37	38	39	40	41	42	43	44	45	46	47	48	49	50	51	52	53	54
Height (inches)	Body Weight (pounds)																		
58	172	177	181	186	191	196	201	205	210	215	220	224	229	234	239	244	248	253	258
59	178	183	188	193	198	203	208	212	217	222	227	232	237	242	247	252	257	262	267
60	184	189	194	199	204	209	215	220	225	230	235	240	245	250	255	261	266	271	276
61	190	195	201	206	211	217	222	227	232	238	243	248	254	259	264	269	275	280	285
62	196	202	207	213	218	224	229	235	240	246	251	256	262	267	273	278	284	289	295
63	203	208	214	220	225	231	237	242	248	254	259	265	270	278	282	287	293	299	304
64	209	215	221	227	232	238	244	250	256	262	267	273	279	285	291	296	302	308	314
65	216	222	228	234	240	246	252	258	264	270	276	282	288	294	300	306	312	318	324
66	223	229	235	241	247	253	260	266	272	278	284	291	297	303	309	315	322	328	334
67	230	236	242	249	255	261	268	274	280	287	293	299	306	312	319	325	331	338	344
68	236	243	249	256	262	269	276	282	289	295	302	308	315	322	328	335	341	348	354
69	243	250	257	263	270	277	284	291	297	304	311	318	324	331	338	345	351	358	365
70	250	257	264	271	278	285	292	299	306	313	320	327	334	341	348	355	362	369	376
71	257	265	272	279	286	293	301	308	315	322	329	338	343	351	358	365	372	379	386
72	265	272	279	287	294	302	309	316	324	331	338	346	353	361	368	375	383	390	397
73	272	280	288	295	302	310	318	325	333	340	348	355	363	371	378	386	393	401	408
74	280	287	295	303	311	319	326	334	342	350	358	365	373	381	389	396	404	412	420
75	287	295	303	311	319	327	335	343	351	359	367	375	383	391	399	407	415	423	431
76	295	304	312	320	328	336	344	353	361	369	377	385	394	402	410	418	426	435	443

Appendix B1
Insurance Letter

Insurance Company
P.O. Box 00000
Dallas, TX 75266-0044

Regarding: Patient:
                Insured:
                Member ID:
                Group No:

Attn: Predetermination

Dear Sir or Madam:

Predetermination/certification of insurance coverage, authorization for hospitalization and surgical treatment are requested on behalf of your annuitant. The patient's general condition, suffering from multiple diagnoses, is complicating the underlying clinically severe disease of **Morbid Obesity [insert insurance code here]**. These conditions typically improve or disappear with weight loss.

This individual is 5'8", weighs 262.5 pounds, and has a body mass index of 40 with co-morbid conditions of hypertension, sleep apnea, and dyslipedemia. She has been severely obese for many years, despite dietary efforts including physician-supervised diet with pills, including Meridian and Fen-phen; non-physician-supervised diets—WeightWatchers; liquid diets including Slim-Fast; miscellaneous diet programs, including low-calorie diets, low-fat diets, high-protein diets, self-imposed fasts, HerbaLife, and Atkins; over-the-counter diet pills, including Metabolife; and health club memberships. She has been unable to achieve a healthful body habitus by dietary restrictions. As pointed out in the NIH Consensus Panel, it is very unlikely that she could accomplish this goal in the future. The scientific facts are that despite years of treatments directed toward long-term reduction of body weight by nonsurgical methods, 90 to 95 percent of persons who lose weight subsequently regain it. It is also well documented that there is significant increase in mortality as the body mass index exceeds 32K/m2. An editorial in the *New England Journal of Medicine* states: "Studies provide additional evidence to strengthen the already compelling conclusion that extreme obesity shortens lives." Studies also show a substantial increase in the risk of diabetes with even a modest weight gain. This is truly a morbid and life-threatening disease.

These conditions predictably will, along with other problems, as they characteristically appear, become increasingly incapacitating in the absence of significant weight loss. Since medical management has failed to produce and maintain weight loss for this patient, I strongly believe bariatric surgery is necessary in order to successfully resolve or ameliorate the multiple medical problems associated with **morbid obesity**.

I am requesting authorization for **an in-patient admission** for a *LAPAROSCOPIC SHORT LIMB (less than 150 cm.) GASTRIC BYPASS* [CODE] to be performed for the treatment of the patient's severe and life-threatening diseases. This procedure will be performed at **The Methodist Hospital** (tax ID #74-1180155) located at 6565 Fannin Street, Houston, TX 77030, 713-790-3311 and an **Assistant Surgeon is required for this procedure.** Without this or a similar procedure, I am certain that significant problems could develop, which will result in future costly hospitalization(s).

It is abundantly clear that the patient meets the requirements set to determine who is a surgical candidate. As I have reviewed all options with the patient, in true informed consent, she has a good understanding of the surgical procedure and complications and has determined that bariatric surgery is the best option for her. Additionally, she understands that the surgery will require lifelong medical observation.

I most strongly request that you clear your annuitant for coverage. Her diseases are progressive and life threatening; I would ask for an efficient and timely review of this case. To require any further "medical" or "dietary" treatment or documentation would be medically unsound and dangerous. Medical treatment is well known to be ineffective, with almost all persons who lose weight regaining it within five years. Should your company therefore require additional dietary attempts, you are in effect requiring the patient to undergo **proven ineffective therapy** before you allow proven treatment regiment—surgery.

Denial of coverage may cause serious injury, or permanent disability, through lack of access to necessary surgical treatment. **Morbid Obesity** has been held by the federal appeals courts to be a disability under the Americans with Disabilities Act. For your annuitant, discrimination against such disability, with respect to provision of contracted medical benefits, may violate the insured's civil rights under that legislation, and may subject the employer or carrier to additional risk.

I am requesting from you, in writing, a preauthorization for inpatient surgery.

Sincerely,

Dr. Garth Davis

Appendix B2

Letter from Your PCP in Support of Your Application

To Whom It May Concern:

Mr./Mrs./Ms. _____ has been a patient of
mine for _____ years. Her weight at each yearly office visit has been:

__/__ Wt:
__/__ Wt:
__/__ Wt:
__/__ Wt:
__/__ Wt:

He/she has done several different diet programs, including:

_____

I have offered instructions on diet at several different visits.

I have also prescribed the following weight-loss meds:

_____

He/she suffers from the following diseases that have been shown to be caused by
or made worse by obesity:

_____

He/she is on the following medications to treat these co-morbidities:

_____

He/she has a family history of obesity as well as a family history of

_____

In my opinion, Mr./Mrs./Ms. _____ is morbidly obese by NIH criteria
and is suffering from co-morbidities of obesity and should therefore be approved
for weight-loss surgery.

Sincerely,

Dr. X

Appendix C
Protein-Rich Foods

Following is a list of popular protein-rich foods:

Protein		
Food	**Amount**	**Grams of protein**
Lean meat (beef, poultry, fish, pork)	1 ounce (by weight)	7
Low-fat cheese	1 ounce (by weight)	7
Tofu (1 ounce)	1 ounce	3–4
Egg • 1 egg (soft-boiled, poached, or scrambled) • 2 egg whites or • ⅛ cup egg substitute	1 ounce (by weight)	7
Milk (skim or 1%) or soy milk	½ cup	4
Non-fat dry milk (dry)	2 tablespoons	4
Low-fat cottage cheese	¼ cup	6
Yogurt (light or plain)	¼ cup	2–3
Beans (kidney, pinto, lentils)	¼ cup	3.5
Vegetables	¼ cup	1
Grains (cereal, pasta, rice)	¼ cup	1.5

Appendix D
Protein Supplements

Supplement Amount /serving	Calories	Protein (grams)	Carbs (grams)	Fat (grams)
Syntrax Nectar *(1 scoop—27 grams)*	90	23	0	0
EAS 100% Whey *(1 scoop—30 grams)*	120	23	3	2
Zero Carb Isopure *(1 bottle—20 fluid ounces)*	160	40	0	0
GNC Pro Performance *(1 scoop—31 grams)*	130	21	5	2.5
Cytosport Complete *(1 scoop—22 grams)*	90	18	1	1.5
Zero Carb Isopure RTD *(1 bottle—20 fluid ounces)*	160	40	0	0
UNJURY *(1 packet—26 grams)*	70	20	3	0
Non-fat dry milk powder *(2 tablespoons—15.3 grams)*	54	8	7.8	0.11
Procel *(1 scoop—6.6 grams)*	28	5	1	0.5
100% Any Whey *(1 scoop—20.5 grams)*	70	17	1	0

Helpful Hints to Get Your Protein Up

1. Add 1 scoop of protein powder to sugar-free instant gelatin or sugar-free pudding mixes.

2. Mix 1 scoop of protein powder into 1 cup of skim or 1% milk 1 to 2 times each day between meals.

3. Add 2 tablespoons of dry non-fat milk powder to any liquid, soup, hot cereal, or skim or 1% milk.

4. Include (at least) 3 to 4 ounces of lean or low-fat meat or meat alternative 3 times each day.

Appendix E
1,400-Calorie Meal Plan

Breakfast:

Choose ONE starch

- ½ cup cereal (hot or cold)
- ½ bagel (1 ounce) or ½ English muffin
- 1 slice toast: whole-wheat or rye
- 1 reduced-fat waffle with 2 tablespoons sugar-free syrup

Choose ONE fruit

- Fresh: 1 small banana, apple, orange, nectarine, or peach, or ¾ cup berries, or 1 cup melon, or ½ cup grapefruit sections
- Canned: ½ cup fruit in natural juices

Choose ONE milk

- 1 cup skim or 1% milk or non-fat or low-fat yogurt (plain or fruit-flavored with aspartame)

Choose ONE meat

- 1 egg
- 1 ounce low-fat cheese

Choose ONE fat

- 1 teaspoon olive, canola, or peanut oil
- 1 tablespoon lower-fat margarine spread

Non-caloric beverages

- 6 to 12 ounces sugar-free drink mix, decaf coffee, or tea or water
- Water intake at least 8 cups daily

Lunch:

Choose ONE starch

- 2 slices of diet bread: whole-wheat or rye (80 calories)
- ½ pita bread or 1 ounce reduced-fat crackers

Choose ONE meat

- 6 ounces skinless chicken/turkey breast, shrimp, tuna (in water), or fat-free cheese
- 4 ounces lean roast beef, ham, or low-fat deli meat

Choose ONE vegetable (raw)

- 2½ cups lettuce, tomato, carrots, celery, cabbage, cucumber, mushrooms, onion, pepper, broccoli, or cauliflower

Choose ONE (fruit)

- Fresh: 1 small banana, apple, orange, nectarine, peach, or ¾ cup berries, or 1 cup melon, or ½ cup grapefruit sections
- Canned: ½ cup fruit in natural juices

Choose ONE fat

- 1 teaspoon olive, canola, or peanut oil
- 1 tablespoon lower-fat margarine spread
- 1 tablespoon salad dressing
- 2 tablespoons reduced-fat salad dressing

Dinner:

Choose TWO starches

- 1 sweet potato, baked or boiled (3 ounces)
- ½ cup cooked whole wheat pasta, rice, corn, peas, or mashed potato
- ½ hot dog or hamburger bun or 1 ounce bread or roll

Choose ONE meat

- 6 ounces fish: flounder, haddock, halibut, cod, or trout
- 6 ounces chicken/turkey breast (skinless), shrimp, scallops, or crab
- 4 ounces lean beef, pork, veal, lamb, or salmon
- 4 ounces lean hamburger patty or reduced-fat hot dog

Choose TWO vegetables

- ½ cup cooked asparagus, beans, broccoli, carrots, cauliflower, spinach, summer squash, tomato sauce, or zucchini
- 1 cup lettuce, tomato, carrots, celery, cabbage, cucumber, mushrooms, onion, pepper, or watercress

Choose ONE fat

- 1 teaspoon olive, canola, or peanut oil
- 1 tablespoon lower-fat margarine spread
- 1 tablespoon salad dressing
- 2 tablespoons reduced-fat salad dressing

Noncaloric beverages

- 6 to 12 ounces sugar-free drink mix, decaf coffee, or tea or water

Snack:

Choose ONE protein
AND
Choose ONE carbohydrate

Protein

- 1 ounce low-fat cheese
- ¼ cup cottage cheese
- 1 tablespoon peanut butter
- ½ cup low-fat plain yogurt

Carbohydrate

- 4 whole-wheat crackers
- ¼ cup pretzels
- 1 small apple or banana
- 15 grapes

Appendix F
Useful Measurement Conversions

3 teaspoons = 1 tablespoon	3 ounces = 1/3 cup
2 tablespoons = 1 ounce	4 ounces = 1/2 cup
1 ounce = 1/8 cup	6 ounces = 3/4 cup
2 ounces = 1/4 cup	8 ounces = 1 cup

Index

About the Authors

Dr. Garth Davis graduated Phi Beta Kappa from the University of Texas in Austin, where he was the student government president. He also received an award as the most outstanding student at UT. He went on to medical school at Baylor College of Medicine and graduated in the top 10 percent of his class, and was inducted to the Alpha Omega Alpha medical honor society. Garth completed his surgical residency at the prestigious University of Michigan, where he was elected to the position of chief administrative resident. While in Michigan, he had extensive experience in general surgical disciplines. He is certified by the American Board of Surgery and is a Fellow of the American College of Surgeons and a Fellow of the American Society for Bariatric Surgery. He has attended many postgraduate courses including laparoscopic and bariatric surgery. He has given several invited lectures on the subject of bariatric surgery.

Garth has had extensive training in laparoscopic surgery and has studied the creation of a full-service integrated weight-loss center. He has specialized in bariatric surgery and is the medical director of the Weight Loss Program at the Methodist Hospital. Garth has been recently recognized as a Texas Monthly Super Doc. He lives in Houston with his family. Visit him at www.thedavisclinic.com.

Laura Tucker is coauthor of books on a wide range of topics. She lives in Brooklyn, New York, with her husband and daughter.